Treating Your MS

A User's Guide to Multiple Sclerosis Medications

STEVEN MANNERS

GARRET EDITIONS
Montreal

Cover design by Éric Théoret, btd-studio.com.

Library and Archives Canada Cataloguing in Publication

Manners, Steven

Treating Your MS: A User's Guide to Multiple Sclerosis Medications / Steven Manners

ISBN 978-0-9878375-3-0

1. Multiple Sclerosis – Medications. 2. Drug development – History.
3. Disease-modifying therapies – Multiple sclerosis. I. Title.

For MBS

Garret Editions

2200 av. Melrose

Montreal, Quebec

Canada H3A 2R8

All inquiries to garreteditions@gmail.com

AVONEX®, TECFIDERA® and FUMADERM® are registered trademarks of Biogen Idec.

TYSABRI® is a registered trademark of Elan Pharma International Ltd.

BETASERON®/BETAFERON® are registered trademarks, used under license by Bayer Inc.

REBIF® is a registered trademark of EMD Serono, Inc.

EXTAVIA* and GILENYA* are registered trademarks of Novartis AG.

COPAXONE® is a registered trademark of Teva Pharmaceutical Industries Ltd.

AUBAGIO® and LEMTRADA® are registered trademarks of Genzyme, a Sanofi company.

Note: The opinions expressed in this book are those of the author and should not be used as the basis for prescribing or self-medication. Consult your health care providers for information specific to your medical condition, and the prescribing information contained in the product monograph for the indications, contraindications and side effects of specific medications. Information is current as of February 2015.

Produced in USA

CONTENTS

INTRODUCTION

IT WAS TWO DECADES AGO that a quiet revolution began in multiple sclerosis. Up until that time, there were no effective treatments to control the disease and little a doctor could do. Then in 1993, the first of the disease-modifying therapies for MS – interferon-beta-1b (Betaseron) – was approved, signalling the beginning of the treatment era. By the end of the first decade, there were two other interferons (Avonex, Rebif) and glatiramer acetate (Copaxone) from which to choose. These so-called ABC drugs (or CRAB after the arrival of Rebif, and BRACE after Extavia) had a few things in common. All needed to be injected. All reduced the frequency of MS relapses (also called attacks or exacerbations). And all had troublesome side effects – flu-like symptoms for the interferons, skin pitting and denting for Copaxone – that made them difficult to take during the life-long course of treatment.

One of the curiosities of first-generation treatments was that they were developed because of misbegotten ideas. Copaxone was originally intended to cause demyelination in an animal model of MS rather than treat MS itself. The interferons targeted a virus that was presumed to cause MS, although such a virus has never been found. But as the virus theory was eclipsed in the 1990s, new ideas came to the fore. MS was seen as an autoimmune disorder characterized by inflammatory flare-ups in the central nervous system (CNS), a view supported by the growing use of magnetic resonance imaging (MRI) that could visually depict the changes in the brain and spinal cord. Less visible, however, was the slow process of neurodegeneration, in which nerve fibres in the CNS were damaged and destroyed. It was this process – acting both as a consequence of inflammation and in parallel to it – that resulted in the progressive disability that is so often a disheartening consequence of MS.

All of the injectable therapies influenced different aspects of the dysregulated immune response seen in MS. However, a shared limitation was their very modest effectiveness: treatment reduced the number of relapses by about one-third. A common misinterpretation is that this means that an individual who is having three relapses a year can expect to have only two relapses a year after starting treatment. But these statistics refer to a population of people rather than to an individual. One hundred people having 300 relapses can expect to see this number reduced to 200 relapses for the group as a whole, with some people becoming relapse-free and others having the same number of relapses (or more) as before. Unfortunately, it's difficult to know who will respond – and impossible to predict who will get the most benefit before a treatment is started. Trial and error with different medications has been the disappointing lot for many people with MS.

The modest reductions in CNS inflammation seen with the first-generation injectables prompted the obvious question: if a little is good, would more be better? Thus began the second generation of MS therapies, which started with the launch of Tysabri (natalizumab) in 2004. Tysabri was the first of the highly targeted MS therapies – a true designer drug developed to combat CNS inflammation. Its success opened the door for other targeted therapies, all of which were initially used for other diseases and repurposed for MS. This group includes Gilenya (fingolimod) and Lemtrada (alemtuzumab), as well as less targeted drugs such as Tecfidera (dimethyl fumarate) and Aubagio (teriflunomide). What these second-generation drugs have in common is they are generally more potent in suppressing inflammation and/or easier to take than the injectable drugs. The hope is that a stronger drug will have a more lasting effect – reducing not only relapses but also minimizing the devastating disability that can occur in MS.

The second-generation drugs will soon be joined by others, considerably broadening the treatment options available to people living with MS. In development are numerous experimental therapies, such as laquinimod, daclizumab, ocrelizumab, ofatumumab, and a host of others. But with this wealth of choices comes three all-important issues that need to be addressed by anyone with MS.

The first issue is whether the benefits of treatment are worth the time, trouble and expense. What will be gained by starting a course of medication?

Secondly, more potent drugs offer the promise of better control of the MS disease process – but this effectiveness is often accompanied by a risk of serious side effects. Is a 50% decrease in relapses (and perhaps less MS disability down the road) worth it if there is a one-in-a-thousand risk of a debilitating brain infection, a heart attack, or a cancer?

Thirdly, how do you make your "informed consent" about treatment as informed as possible? In the first decade of MS therapies, over 12,000 scientific articles were published on MS. Over the past decade that number has more than doubled to over 25,000 articles (and a four-fold increase in 2012 compared to 1993). How can you keep abreast of all of this research to make the best decision about your treatment plan?

This book is intended to help answer some of your questions about the treatment options available to you. After summarizing what is known about the MS disease process, we'll discuss how different treatments work, what clinical studies have (and haven't) shown, and the benefits and risks of therapy. In the final chapter we'll review some of the issues to consider when deciding on your best approach to controlling your MS.

There is no recipe, no one-size-fits-all, when it comes to treating MS. And a unique aspect of MS care is the amount of input people have in choosing a therapy. Although this will surely shift as treatment options become more complex, it is still important to be aware of what treatments can and can't do and what risks are involved. *Treating Your MS* will guide you through these complexities by summarizing what medical research has uncovered. We'll look at the studies that have been done, and along the way we'll explore some of the ideas that drive MS research so you'll understand the rationale behind therapy.

The approach of the book is to look at the science behind the therapies and present the facts as they're known. But the usual caveat applies: medicine is an evolution of ideas, as answers are sought for specific questions. But the number of questions will always exceed the number of answers, and each answer may in turn open up new lines of inquiry. This idea, that the concepts that drive MS are continually being revised (and sometimes discredited) as new information becomes available, can be unsettling to some. Much about the MS story will become clearer in the future, but people must act in the present. So all you can do is make the best choices today with the most up-to-date information available, while always remaining aware that the plan may need to be modified in the future.

Most people diagnosed with an illness will seek out some information, but the amount that's needed is very much a personal decision. To some, information is only useful to address practical problems: what symptoms to expect, what side effects can happen with which drugs, and so on. Others will want to know more. In part this is a reflection of personal coping style: information can empower or disempower. The goal of *Treating Your MS* is to provide you with what you need to help you cope better with your illness, not to overwhelm you with the details – but the details are there for those who want them. The hope is that you'll be left feeling better able to make an informed decision about the wisest course of action in your personal struggle against MS.

Part I

THE MS DISEASE PROCESS

CHAPTER 1

WHAT IS MS?

PERHAPS THE MOST COMMON QUESTION a person has when first diagnosed with multiple sclerosis is: *What is MS?* It's also one of the most difficult to answer. Over the years, different ideas about the cause(s) of MS have evolved from various observations to create something that is more like a jigsaw puzzle (with some pieces missing) than a complete picture. These observations come primarily from researchers studying in laboratories, doctors treating individual patients, investigators in large clinical trials, and analyses of large databases of MS patients.

What they have learned thus far can be summarized in an oft-repeated phrase: MS is believed to be an autoimmune disorder caused by a complex interaction of genetic and environmental factors. The sentence incorporates three separate but overlapping ideas – the immune system, genetics and the environment – and each needs its own explanation. So in this chapter we'll look at each of these things and how they interact with one another so we can work toward more of a unified picture of MS.

How does the immune system work?

MOST LIVING THINGS, including animals, fish, insects and plants, have an immune system. This so-called innate immune system provides a basic defence against infection by foreign invaders, such as bacteria, viruses and fungi (collectively called pathogens). The first line of defence consists of physical barriers, such as the skin, and the cells lining the respiratory and gastrointestinal tracts. What all but one of these barriers have in common is that they're in direct contact with the outside world through touching, breathing and eating. The sole exception is the physical barrier that protects the brain. The blood vessels that enter the brain are lined with a layer of tightly-packed cells called the blood-brain barrier (BBB). The BBB acts like a wall, protecting the inner fortress of the brain from harmful substances. This wall has gates to allow necessary supplies (such as nutrients) to be transported in, and waste materials (the result of the brain's metabolic activities) to be transported out.

The second line of defence is the immune response, which involves specialized cells that fulfill three main functions. The first task is to detect Stranger or Danger.[1] The Strangers are pathogens that cause disease, and other foreign substances (e.g. pollen, toxins) that might harm the body. The Dangers are problems such as tissue damage caused by injury, or abnormal cells, such as cancer cells. Once a problem is detected, the second function of immunity is to launch an immune attack, which involves walling off the area to contain the hot spot, calling for back-up from other immune cells, and destroying any pathogens or damaged tissue. Once this is accomplished, the third function is to mop up, removing the debris and repairing the damage. All of these processes are at work with something as simple as cutting your finger. The finger becomes red and swollen as the area is flooded with immune cells, pus forms (from dead immune cells and pathogens), the damage is repaired, and the cut heals.

The immune system in humans is actually two systems that act in parallel. The innate immune response is very ancient and its great advantage is that it acts very quickly. The disadvantage is that it's not very fine-tuned. It's a police officer walking a beat and watching for signs of trouble rather than a highly specialized SWAT team. Innate immune cells are always patrolling the body but they don't really know what they're looking for. So they "profile" using pattern recognition. The profiles they recognize are suspicious molecules belonging to pathogens, or from damaged cells in your body.

The limitations of the innate immune system leave room for improvement. So higher animals (those with a backbone and a jawbone) have evolved a second system of defence, called the adaptive immune system. As the name implies, this immune response adapts itself in response to the pathogens it encounters. Since adaptive immunity can recognize a pathogen it has seen before (the idea behind vaccination), it can respond in a much more targeted way to fight disease. This adaptability makes a person's immune system unlike anyone else's because part of its makeup consists of past experiences. This has been called the "biography" of the immune system.[2]

MS is generally considered to be a dysfunction of the adaptive immune response. Three key players in this scenario are specialized immune cells called B cells (which are produced in the bone marrow); T cells (because they mature in the thymus located behind your breast bone); and antigen-presenting cells (APCs), which describes a function rather than a specific type of cell. B cells and T cells are types of white blood cells (called lymphocytes) that travel along the two main highways of the body – the blood stream and the lymphatic system – looking for problem antigens. An antigen is any substance that triggers an antibody response; it may be parts of a bacterium or virus, but it may also be grass pollen, bee venom, different foods, and so on.

While the innate immune system profiles, the acquired immune system uses a Stop and Frisk approach (to continue the policing analogy). In the case of B cells, they bind to bits of what they find in their environment (these bits are proteins, fats or complex sugars). This binding of the B cell to a substance is not unlike running an electronic passkey through a reader. If the substance doesn't have the right code, the B cell becomes activated. Its response is to produce antibodies that are specific to the foreign substance. Producing antibodies is just one way a B cell can respond. A B cell can also fulfill the role of an APC by ingesting ("eating") the substance. This allows it to "present" the antigen on its cell surface, with the antigen appearing like a hotdog sticking out from a hotdog bun. Other types of APCs include macrophages ("big eaters") and dendritic cells, both components of the older innate immune system.

T cells differ from B cells in that they can't bind to antigens directly. They need to be presented with the offending substance by an APC. As part of this process, APCs bind the antigen to a molecule called Major Histocompatibility Complex (MHC) (also called human leukocyte antigen or HLA). You may be familiar with HLA from "tissue typing" for organ transplantation. We can think of the MHC molecule as an ID badge that is used to display the name of the antigen. The T cell's job is to check the ID. If the antigen fails the check, the T cell becomes activated and starts an immune reaction. As part of the collaboration of T and B cells, a T-cell response will also amplify the B cell's ability to produce more antibodies. But T cells also act on their own. When they detect a specific antigen, they quickly expand their own numbers. The result is a large population of T cells, all primed to respond to that very specific antigen that initiated the response. This enables the immune response to be highly directed at one particular problem.

As part of this specific response, T cells will develop into one of several types. These types have somewhat different buttons that get pushed to release different chemical messengers, which then communicate in different ways with other cells. You may be unaccustomed to the idea that a chemical can act as a form of communication, but this is common throughout nature. The scent trail that an ant leaves enables it to communicate with other ants. Hormones and perfumes also act as chemical signals. In fact, interferon (one of the MS treatments we'll discuss) is a type of cytokine, or chemical signal, naturally produced by cells in the body.

Among the various types of T cells that can develop, of particular importance to MS are T-helper cells (Th). When a Th cell responds to a stimulus, it may promote inflammation (a Th1 response) or it may be anti-inflammatory (a Th2 response). In recent years, two additional subtypes have been shown to play an important role in MS.

Th17 cells promote inflammation and appear to be especially damaging to tissues. Regulatory T cells (Tregs) act to moderate the immune (and autoimmune) response, shutting down the inflammatory process and returning the immune system back to a quiescent state.

What happens in MS?

SO WHAT GOES WRONG IN MS?

If we think of the immune response as a home alarm system, several things can go wrong and the consequences may be dramatic. Suppose you enter your passcode but the alarm goes off anyway. The police arrive and mistake you for an intruder, kicking down your door and damaging your home in the process. This is essentially what happens in MS.

The main culprit in MS is believed to be the T cell. In checking the ID badges presented by APCs, T cells are supposed to be able to tell the difference between Stranger/Danger antigens and Self antigens (i.e. substances from your own body). Indeed, as they mature in the thymus, T cells that are too autoreactive (i.e. shown to respond to the body's own antigens) are quickly destroyed (the same happens to autoreactive B cells). But in MS, T cells mistake Self for Stranger and become activated. The underlying problem may be that as T cells were developing, the bad T cells (the autoreactive ones) weren't weeded out. Or the problem may be a hidden flaw in some T cells, which causes them to get switched on when they were supposed to stay switched off.

The problem is then compounded as this T-cell population quickly expands in number. As mentioned before, T cells are highly targeted. When a specific T cell finds a specific problem, its response is to divide very rapidly to produce more of itself. So the result is a large population of T cells patrolling the body looking for that specific antigen. This is what's needed if the antigen is a type of bacteria – you want to remove every trace of the disease. But a problem arises if the antigen is a substance in your own body. The immune system launches an attack, which results in inflammation and tissue damage wherever that antigen is found in the body.

In the case of autoimmune disorders, the immune response doesn't protect the body – it attacks certain tissues in the body, depending on the type of disorder. In Type 1 (juvenile) diabetes, the immune attack is directed at the cells in the pancreas that produce insulin. In rheumatoid arthritis or lupus, the immune attack is largely directed at connective tissue in the joints.

In MS, the target of the immune attack is myelin, the fatty tissue that covers nerve fibres in the CNS. This myelin acts as an insulator for the electrical "wiring" of the nerve fibre, enabling nerve signals to be transmitted more efficiently and more rapidly. T cells that have become reactive to one of the constituents of myelin go off in search of it. The prime source of myelin is in the CNS, so these activated T cells cross the blood-brain barrier and enter the brain and spinal cord, where they cause inflammation and tissue damage. As the "insulation" protecting nerve fibres is eroded, the electrical signals passing along the nerves get interrupted. These short circuits are then experienced as MS symptoms. The type of symptom reflects the part of the CNS that's affected and the types of neurons that are experiencing damage. So damaged sensory nerves will cause tingling, numbness or nerve pain; damaged optic nerves will cause vision problems; damaged motor (muscle) nerves will cause muscle rigidity, weakness or bowel/bladder problems; and so on. All of this takes place in the brain. You may feel that the nerves in your numb hand are affected but those peripheral nerves are intact. The problem originates in messages from the brain.

So this is the simplified three-part scheme of the autoimmune reaction in MS:

1. T cells become abnormally activated in response to Self antigens.

2. T cells cross the blood-brain barrier and enter the CNS.

3. T cells then initiate and sustain an immune response in the brain and spinal cord that causes demyelination (loss of myelin) and damage to nerve fibres.

THE CENTRAL ROLE THAT T CELLS PLAY in the disease process is reflected in the therapies that have been developed to treat MS. All of them target this T-cell response in one way or another. However, this simplified scheme doesn't fully capture all of the nuances of the immune response or the complexities of the disease. For example, there is extensive cross-talk between T cells and B cells, so a number of new therapies in development are now targeting the B-cell response.

The sequence of events is also unduly focused on what is happening in the body rather than what is happening in the CNS – and MS is ultimately a disease of the brain, spinal cord and optic nerve. So this raises an important question: does MS start in the body or in the brain?

This is a highly controversial question. The prevailing theory about the beginnings of MS is the Outside-in Model: T cells become activated outside the CNS, then migrate into the CNS to cause inflammation and damage.

However, some have speculated that MS is an Inside-Out disease. In other words, the immune system is actually responding to a problem in the brain, and other immune players (such as T and B cells) are summoned into the brain to help with the problem. If this is true, it raises the question of what is the problem in the CNS, and there has been a great deal of speculation about this. It may be that there's an inbuilt defect in the myelin. The brain's own immune response tries to fix the damage by cleaning up the myelin debris, in effect "presenting" myelin as a problem antigen. It may be that the myelin is not inherently defective but has been damaged by a pathogen, such as a virus. Or there may be that native immune cells in the brain switch on and stay switched on, which ultimately leads to "hot spots" of inflammation and damage.

One of the more fanciful ideas derives from the Human Genome Project, which has been mapping the sequence of human genes. One finding was that many genes – about 8% of our genetic code – aren't human in origin. They originated from viruses. During our evolution as a species, these viral genes were so useful to our cellular machinery (and obviously not lethal) that we borrowed them and put them to work. To put this into perspective, the finding that people of non-African descent had some Neanderthal genes caused a bit of a stir – but viral genes in the human genome are twice as common as Neanderthal genes. These viral genes may or may not be expressed; they may be switched on and off as the need arises. So one theory is that if a viral gene periodically switches on and produces viral proteins, this might trigger an immune response in a pattern similar to the immune activation that's seen in MS. This idea is now being explored in a trial of antiviral therapy in MS and that should help to determine if this notion has any merit. We'll look more at viruses as a possible trigger for MS later on in this chapter.

What happens to the central nervous system in MS?

WHEN T CELLS INVADE THE CNS, they promote an inflammatory response that erodes the myelin insulation that protects nerve fibres, a process called demyelination. These pockets of inflammation are seen as discrete lesions on magnetic resonance imaging (MRI). Some of this damage can be repaired by specialized brain cells that produce myelin (called oligodendrocytes). However, the process of remyelination may be incomplete or flawed so that the nerve fibre remains exposed. Remyelination may fail because there's just too much damage to repair, or the inflammatory environment is too toxic for the process to be completed.

A stripped nerve fibre may continue to function but it's like a bare wire that suffers interruptions ("sparks"), which are experienced as nerve symptoms (tingling, numbness, pain or weakness). Inflammation doesn't directly kill off the nerve fibre. But that nerve fibre will die if it experiences a "second hit". What that second hit may be is a matter of some speculation. One idea is that there may be a defect in the mitochondria. This are specialized organs within a cell and one of their functions is to be an energy source; in effect, they are the batteries (and even resemble AA batteries) that allow cells to function. So the nerve fibre may experience a "brown out". Another theory involves the ion channels that propagate electrical signals along the nerve. Dysregulation of this process may essentially cause an "overload" which kills the nerve fibre.

Inflammation is usually a self-regulating process, so why doesn't this inflammatory response shut down? Many conditions, such as infections, head trauma or stroke, will cause damage to the CNS. And yet this damage doesn't result in a widespread and sustained inflammatory response. MS is quite different in that regard, and it may be that there's a defect in how the body cleans up the bits of damaged myelin – in effect, mistaking these bits as "foreign" antigen, which then fuels the fire and sustains the reaction. It may be that the T cells (called regulatory T cells, or Tregs) that are supposed to modulate and shut down the immune reaction are not up to the job.

Another notion is that the initial T cell response induces cells in the brain (e.g. astrocytes and microglia[3,4]) to become activated, resulting in more widespread inflammation. This is a hot topic in MS research today. Until recently, researchers were primarily interested in the focal inflammatory lesions that are a key characteristic of MS. In part this was because these lesions are highly visible on an MRI. What is harder to detect on MRI is more diffuse inflammation throughout the brain, which probably contributes to much of the neurodegeneration and tissue loss that occurs in progressive MS. This neurodegeneration is what underlies the disabilities that occur later on in the disease process, so it's a key target – and arguably the most important target – for treatment. Some of the current MS medications may have an impact on diffuse inflammation (such as Gilenya, Tecfidera and Aubagio), and a number of newer therapies are being expressly developed to try to reduce the loss of nerve fibres in the brain.

What triggers MS?

THUS FAR WE'VE SEEN that the central idea behind MS is a problem with the T cell response: it's a case of mistaken identity and the error becomes magnified without the immune system re-establishing control. The mistaken identity comes when a T cell scans an antigen's ID badge and responds as if one of the body's myelin proteins is something foreign. But why does this mistake happen?

To explain this we need to introduce the idea of "molecular mimicry". As the term implies, one molecule can resemble (or mimic) another molecule. When a foreign antigen is presented to a T cell, the T cell population expands and goes in search of this same antigen. If the foreign antigen is a protein fragment – just a short sequence of amino acids – it may closely resemble other amino acid sequences. After all, there are only 22 standard amino acids and a finite number of permutations and combinations with which to make up a protein fragment.

This is where viruses enter the story. Throughout the 1980s, a prevailing concept was that MS was caused by a virus. As recently as two decades ago, one of the modern pioneers of MS research, John Kurtzke (of the eponymous Kurtzke Expanded Disability Status Scale, or EDSS), thought that MS was actually an infectious disease.[5] This belief was held by many and fuelled the investigation of antiviral medications for MS in the 1980s, a time when viruses (herpes, HIV) were the focus of a great deal of medical research. As a further spur to this activity, new techniques were developed in the 1980s that enabled the mass production of "biologicals" through recombinant DNA technology. Among the first drugs to be developed using these techniques were two that would later become MS therapies: alemtuzumab (now called Lemtrada), and the interferons (Avonex, Betaseron/Extavia and Rebif). The interferons are now believed to work in MS through mechanisms that have little or nothing to do with their antiviral properties, but the virus theory of MS has persisted in one form or another to this day.

Whether MS is an autoimmune disorder or a viral disease is a matter of some dispute. However, it may not be a question of either/or: MS may be triggered by a virus and the disease course may be maintained through autoimmune-like mechanisms. But just to clarify, when people talk about viruses as the trigger for MS, they don't mean that the signs and symptoms of MS are necessarily caused by an infection. One theory is that you may have encountered a virus at some point. That virus may or may not have caused an illness (some viruses don't), but your immune system successfully contained it. "Contained" rather than killed, since some viruses, such as the herpesvirus that causes chickenpox or the JC virus that causes progressive multifocal leukoencephalopathy (PML), are never cleared from your body. The immune system suppresses them and they go into hiding. And like a sleeper cell, they can be reactivated if the body ever lets down its guard. In the case of chickenpox (varicella zoster), the virus can flare up and cause painful shingles later in life.

After your immune system has encountered a virus, it learns how to recognize certain viral antigens. This virus is now part of your immune biography, and your immune system will respond quickly if it detects this virus again. This is why people are vaccinated – so their immune system can learn to recognize a specific disease-causing organism.

What the immune system recognizes are specific antigens from the virus. If that sequence becomes altered – if the virus changes its appearance – then the immune system won't recognize it and won't be able to mobilize its defences against it. An example is the common cold – caused by a virus that changes its appearance so quickly that any vaccine would soon be out of date. More recently, the antigens in the flu vaccine developed for the 2014-2015 winter season were not the best assortment so the vaccine wasn't especially effective.

But what if the viral antigen resembles other antigens – such as antigens (i.e. a certain amino acid sequence) from your own body? As the immune system does its Stop and Frisk, it can start "arresting" too many things that only resemble what it's looking for. An example of this is hepatitis B. A protein from hepatitis B is very similar to myelin basic protein (MBP), one of the components of myelin, and an immune response to one carries over to the other.[6,7]

The viral trigger that's most often cited as a candidate is Epstein-Barr virus (EBV), which causes mononucleosis (the "kissing disease").

Most people encounter this virus at some point in their lives. This is shown by antibodies to EBV, which are detectable in over 90% of the adult population – but even more commonly among people with MS.[8,9] Most people develop an EBV infection in infancy or childhood, often without knowing it. When EBV is encountered later in life, it can manifest as mononucleosis. This is a curious feature of our immune biography – that the timing of an infection can determine how a disease develops. An infection during childhood is often more severe than if you contracted the illness later in life because your immune system is less capable of fighting it. But the reverse is also true: some illnesses that are generally mild in childhood (such as mumps) can cause serious complications if you contract them as an adult.

Since most people are exposed to EBV, it makes it very difficult to determine if the virus is an actual cause of MS. Some have suggested that an EBV infection after puberty increases the risk of MS,[10] others that a one-two punch of EBV and another mystery virus are behind it all.[11] (The mystery virus was never identified although it did acquire a name, MS-associated virus,[12] which managed to sound specific and nonspecific at the same time.) The suggestion was that people who got "mono" in adolescence or early adulthood were more likely to develop MS many years later.[13] Other infections after age 15, such as measles or mumps, may also be important.[14] However, while many studies have suggested that EBV is involved somehow in the development of MS,[15,16] the precise nature of that involvement is still a matter of speculation.

It's possible that EBV is only one of several viruses, acting alone or in concert with other pathogens, that can induce an abnormal immune response in susceptible people. One problem in sorting out these complexities is that the actual trigger – a specific viral antigen – hasn't been found.

Researchers still hope to identify a specific virus that causes MS, but it may not matter that much. This is because of another idea that we need to introduce, called "epitope spreading", first described two decades ago.[17] When APCs (such as macrophages or dendritic cells) digest protein fragments, the antigen they display is just one of many. The antigen component that a T cell recognizes is called an epitope, but any number of a fistful of epitopes in the protein may be displayed. So as the T cell reacts to one epitope, it may also react to other epitopes in that cluster. In this way, a highly specific immune response can become less specific. This may make sense if the antigen is part of a virus protein – it would be a good strategy to learn to recognize other components of that virus. But if there's mistaken identity, epitope spreading only makes the problem worse. It becomes a case of broken telephone: a viral antigen is mistaken for one type of myelin protein (e.g. myelin oligodendrocyte glycoprotein, or MOG), which in turn is mistaken for another type of myelin protein (e.g. myelin basic protein [MBP] or proteolipid protein [PLP]). This chain of events has been shown in animal models. In mice infected with a virus, microglia in the brain respond to the infection by presenting the viral antigen to T cells; the T cells react to a specific myelin protein; and then the T cells start to react to additional myelin proteins,[18] so that the immune reaction becomes a more widespread and more damaging inflammatory response.

In practical terms, what this sequence of events means is that by the time someone is diagnosed with MS, their body is reacting to a wide range of Self antigens so there probably isn't a specific antigen (viral or otherwise) that is causing the problem. This may explain why MS symptoms worsen during a viral infection (such as the flu):[19] a new dose of virus may add fuel to the fire by providing the immune system with more antigen. It may also be the reason that antiviral medications, such as Zovirax (acyclovir) or Valtrex (valacyclovir), haven't been effective in treating MS.[20-22] By the time treatment is used to target a specific virus, the problem has become too widespread for the medication to do any good. Ceiling sprinklers will do little to control a fire if the roof is already ablaze.

Why me?

WHY DOES MS DEVELOP in some people and not others? Why is it more common in certain populations, such as Caucasians of European ancestry, and less common in others, such as Asians or African blacks? Differences in populations raises the issue of genetics. MS is not a "genetic disease" in which a specific mutation that you are born with (as in cystic fibrosis) or which you acquire (as in chronic myeloid leukemia) actually causes an illness. Rather, slight genetic variations are believed to contribute to the risk of MS, although how that occurs is largely unknown. The main problem is that the cause of MS hasn't been identified, so it isn't possible to identify a specific gene that contributes to the development of MS.

Since MS is believed to be an autoimmune disorder, much of the research into the genetics of MS has focused on genes that code for different aspects of the immune response. T cells are considered to be the main culprits, but they don't function on their own. To recognize and react to antigens, T cells must have the antigen presented to them. As we've seen, this service is performed by APCs, which bind antigen to a molecule called major histocompatibility complex (MHC, also known as human leukocyte antigen, or HLA). You may be familiar with HLA from "tissue typing", i.e. matching a donor to a recipient for organ transplantation. HLA genes are the most varied of any in the human genome, which means that they are evolving and changing more rapidly than other genes. This variability enables a population to meet the challenge of the wide range of pathogens that the MHC may encounter. Slightly different versions of these genes (called alleles) will produce slightly different MHC molecules, which will then act a bit differently. This broadens the human response to disease – a good survival strategy when a population is exposed to a new epidemic. However, this variability can also cause problems. In fact, many autoimmune disorders (such as Type 1 diabetes, lupus and rheumatoid arthritis) are associated with variations in one or more of the HLA genes that produce MHC.

Of particular importance to MS is an HLA gene called *DRB1*, which is responsible for producing a component of the MHC class-II molecule. *DRB1* in some form is found in everyone, but variations of the gene occur with different frequencies in the human population. One variation is the *DRB1*1501* allele.[23] This occurs with high frequency (about 60%[24]) in Caucasian populations and less frequently in other ethnic groups[25] – which may explain in part why MS is more common in whites.

This doesn't mean that *DRB1*1501* is the "MS gene". What it confers is a susceptibility. But it's important to keep in mind that this allele is neither necessary nor sufficient: a person can develop MS without this gene (although they may need another type of genetic variation), and having this allele on its own doesn't mean you will inevitably develop MS. For example, *DRB1*1501* generally isn't found in people with MS in Iran.[26] In Sicily, as in the rest of Italy, *DRB1*1501* is common but other, entirely different HLA alleles, also play a role in MS.[27] With some alleles it's hard to tell if they're friend or foe. An HLA allele (called *DQB1*0602*) is associated with a higher MS risk in whites as well as in blacks from Martinique, African-Americans and Latin Americans.[28-30] But this same allele doesn't seem to be associated with MS in people from the Middle East or Asia.

What all of these *HLA* genes have in common is that they produce different components of the MHC molecule. These small variations may cause the MHC to present antigen to T cells in a slightly different way. The difference may be miniscule, and it's not enough on its own to actually cause MS. But it may be enough to create a susceptibility – provided other factors also come into play. This "multifactorial" model is also seen in other medical conditions: hypertension alone may not cause a stroke, but coupled with genetic factors (e.g. how you process cholesterol) and environmental factors (e.g. smoking), all can act together to increase the risk of stroke.

So genetic and environmental factors may combine to increase a person's risk of developing MS. And other factors (such as sun exposure and smoking) may add to that risk. But genetics alone are not enough. This is seen in twin studies. An identical twin of someone with MS (i.e. with the same genetics) doesn't invariably develop MS – only about 3 in 10 will,[31] which is far less frequent than if MS were a true genetic disease.

How do risk factors interact to cause MS?

THUS FAR WE'VE SEEN THAT VIRUSES such as EBV have been theorized to act as a trigger for MS, and that genetic factors – such as how the immune system presents antigen to T cells – also seem to contribute to the risk of developing MS. Genetic and environmental factors (nature and nurture) don't act in a vacuum, of course – they interact with one another. There's evidence to suggest that the heightened response to EBV is greatest in people with MS if they have the "MS allele" (i.e. *HLA-DRB1*1501*).[32] So this fits with the idea that genetic factors alter how the body responds to viral infection, although it isn't clear how this abnormal response to EBV (or other antigens) actually works.

A fascinating aspect of the altered immune response is the suggestion that there are specific time points in a person's life when infections are especially important. Childhood is a critical time because this is when people first encounter various viruses and bacteria in the environment and their immune system learns how to fight off infections. From an immune standpoint, it's good for children to be exposed to a wide range of pathogens (assuming the diseases aren't life-threatening) because this will broaden their immune system's repertoire – the ability to combat a wide array of different bugs. Conversely, the immune system repertoire will be limited if the child lives in too sterile an environment. (This argument has been used against the widespread use of antibacterial products in the home.)

This part of the MS story is called the "Hygiene Hypothesis"[33] – a much-debated topic in MS research and often put forth as a reason why MS (as well as other autoimmune and allergic disorders) are on the increase worldwide. One of the origins of the hygiene hypothesis in MS is the observation of a "latitude effect" – that MS is increasingly common as you move farther away from the equator. So MS is much more common in Canada or northern Europe than it is in Africa or South America. One way of explaining the latitude effect has been to point to differing levels of hygiene – that children in developing countries have greater exposure to a wide variety of environmental pathogens at an earlier age than kids in more developed countries. This theory is a bit freighted by first-world anxiety about an unnatural, overprocessed environment. But it is supported by the observation that children with younger brothers or sisters are less likely to have an altered immune response to EBV – and less likely to develop MS.[34] That same study found that for children with the highest exposure to a sibling during childhood, the risk of developing MS in later life was reduced by almost 80%. A separate study found that the risk of MS was lower in people who had two or more older siblings, attended daycare or lived in a larger population area – all factors that increase a person's exposure to other people's bugs.[35]

Another critical time is just before MS symptoms develop, which for most people is in their twenties or early thirties. A U.S. analysis of more than three million blood samples found that the antibody response to EBV was similar for everyone up until the age of 20. But by age 25, the antibody response was significantly different among people who later developed MS.[36] Other studies have pointed to the five-year period immediately preceding the development of MS symptoms as being especially important.[37] So it may be that there's an early defect that only manifests later in life. Perhaps this hidden defect only reveals itself if there's a later infection (in adolescence). Or it could be that a few years are needed (or additional events) before a hidden problem comes to light.

The Hygiene Hypothesis is one way of explaining the latitude effect. Another theory points to the differing amounts of sunlight to which people are exposed in various parts of the world. In fact, if you were to plot MS cases on a world map, the result would match up pretty well with a map of the regional exposure to ultraviolet (UV) radiation (i.e. sunlight).[38] This has been done for the United States.[39] States with the lowest UV index, such as Washington, Minnesota or New Hampshire have a six-fold higher incidence of MS than the sunniest states, such as Florida or New Mexico. The same holds true for France: MS is much more common in the northwest city of Rouen compared to the French Riviera.[40]

Sun exposure has also been used to explain the month-of-birth effect in MS. In Canada and northern Europe, MS is significantly more common in people born in the month of May and less common in people born in November.[41,42] A May birth corresponds to when a pregnant woman has her lowest amount of sun exposure, whereas for a November birth there is the highest sun exposure. (The reverse would be true for the southern hemisphere.) However, the importance of this observation is unclear. A recent study has argued that there is no month-of-birth effect: it's simply that in northern latitudes, more babies are born in the spring and summer,[43] so inevitably more babies are born who will later develop MS.

Differences in sun exposure drew researchers' attention to vitamin D. This vitamin (actually a hormone) is called the "sunshine vitamin" because that's how it originates. When skin is exposed to sunlight it produces vitamin D from a cholesterol-type molecule (called 7-dehydrocholesterol). This chemical reaction occurs because of ultraviolet-B (UV-B); it can also occur to a lesser degree after exposure to a tanning bed, which uses mostly UV-A radiation. The chemical reaction results in the formation of vitamin D3 (also known as cholecalciferol). To become biologically active, vitamin D3 must be converted to calcitriol (often abbreviated as 1,25[OH]D) in the kidneys and immune cells.

Vitamin D is important because of its role in bone metabolism: a vitamin D deficiency in childhood causes rickets. But vitamin D is also involved in regulating immune function. As long ago as 1960, researchers speculated that MS was related in some way to sunshine.[44] In keeping with this idea, it may be that MS is becoming increasingly common in part because of the more widespread use of sun-blocking agents. Thus far, research has found that people with MS have fewer relapses after taking vitamin D supplements.[45] Experiments have also shown that vitamin D can inhibit immune system activation by suppressing the types of T cells implicated in MS,[46] and to slow progression in an animal model of MS.[47]

Once vitamin D has been converted to a biologically active form in the body, it acts on various tissues via a specialized receptor called the vitamin D receptor (or VDR). VDRs are found on many cells in the immune system, including T cells, B cells and macrophages.[48-50] So vitamin D can suppress the activation of T cells; shift the immune response to a less inflammatory profile; and induce regulatory T cells to modulate the immune response. It has been suggested that vitamin D acts on the immune system's feedback loop to dampen the damaging effects of inflammation, in part by reducing the proliferation of B cells.[51]

So vitamin D would appear to have the potential to quieten some of the immune system overactivity seen in MS. It's a fine theory, but one that is still waiting to be proven. Clinical studies have failed to show that taking vitamin D supplements has much of an impact on MS. Thus far, only two small trials have been completed and both failed to show a benefit with vitamin D supplements. In the first study, people took either a lower dose (1000 IU/day) or a higher dose (6000 IU/day) of vitamin D.[52] Most were taking either a beta-interferon or glatiramer acetate for their MS. While the higher dose resulted in higher blood levels of vitamin D, it was also associated with worsening disability. There was no difference between the groups with respect to changes on MRI. During the 6-month study, there were four relapses in the high-dose group and none in the lower dose group. One problem with the study was that the supplement was vitamin D2 (ergocalciferol), which is derived from plants. Vitamin D2 and D3 are often thought to be the same, but they have somewhat different effects in the body. Vitamin D3, which is becoming the preferred form in vitamin supplements, has been estimated to be about 3-10 times more potent than vitamin D2 and is more effective at increasing vitamin levels in the bloodstream.[53]

The second study examined the effect of very high doses of vitamin D3 (300,000 IU per month) in 62 people with MS in Iran.[54] After six months of treatment, there was no impact on MRI lesions or disease progression, although immune system activity appeared to be somewhat less in people taking supplements.

Despite these findings, many doctors will recommend vitamin D simply because it may provide some benefit, it's inexpensive and the risks are minimal. The optimal dose of vitamin D hasn't been established, but many groups have recommended anywhere from 800 IU/day up to 2000-4000 IU per day.

AS IN ANY COMPLEX SEQUENCE OF EVENTS, it's difficult to ascertain what is the initiating event, and what are all of the ramifications of the process. There may be an inbuilt error in the body's ability to eliminate self-reactive immune cells, faulty presentation of antigen to T cells by MHC Class II molecules, or a problem in re-establishing normal immune function after a flare-up. There may be additional, subtle differences in how well an individual is able to remyelinate damaged myelin and restore normal signalling in the CNS.

All of these unknowns add up to the key uncertainties of MS: how severe will it be, how long will it take to develop and how much disability will there be. Just as genetic, immune and environmental factors contribute to the development of MS, it's reasonable to assume that genetic, immune and environmental factors will determine the course that MS will take. We'll look at how MS evolves in the next chapter.

One obvious consequence of all of the unknowns is that it's very difficult to develop a medication that will specifically target the problem(s). On a more positive note, such a complex chain of events provides numerous ways for medications to intercede in the disease process. An important shortcoming, however, it that it's unclear which is the right target, or even if there is a right target. So therapies have pursued different approaches.

The target for most MS therapies is the T cell. Some drugs (e.g. interferons, Copaxone) try to shift the T cell response to a less inflammatory profile. Other drugs block activated T cells from entering the brain (e.g. Tysabri), or limit the pool of T cells that is available to attack the CNS (Gilenya). Newer drugs have broader suppressive effects on T and B cells (Lemtrada) or specifically target B cells (ocrelizumab, ofatumumab). How MS therapies act on different aspects of the immune response will be examined in greater detail in Part II.

CHAPTER 2

HOW DOES MS DEVELOP?

THE FOCUS OF THIS BOOK IS ON MS TREATMENTS, but it's important to know how MS evolves during the course of disease. So over the next two chapters we'll look at the earliest stage of MS – which is called clinically isolated syndrome suggestive of MS, or CIS – as well as what's been learned from MS population studies.

How is MS diagnosed?

MS IS A CLINICAL DIAGNOSIS. This means that the diagnosis is based in part on the symptoms a person describes and how long they've had them. The other basis for the diagnosis is what the doctor determines during the neurological exam, which involves testing reflexes and coordination, sensation, movements and balance. The main "paraclinical" tests that may be used to support the diagnosis are lumbar puncture (spinal tap), which checks the cerebrospinal fluid for signs of immune activation in the CNS; and magnetic resonance imaging (MRI), which may reveal inflammatory lesions in the brain and spinal cord that have the appearance or distribution characteristic of MS.

Specific criteria are needed to enable doctors to say with reasonable certainty that a person has MS rather than some other neurological condition (there are literally about 100 conditions that resemble the signs and symptoms of MS). The criteria used to diagnose MS have changed over the years, largely because of the more widespread use of MRI. This new approach was reflected in guidelines published in 2001 that became known as the McDonald criteria after the lead author of the paper, the New Zealand neurologist W. Ian McDonald.[1] The key idea was that MS lesions needed to show "dissemination in space" and "dissemination in time." The "space" requirement means that lesions are affecting more than one area of the CNS. This is easier to see with an MRI but it can be done without a scan by a careful neurological exam; the type of neurological signs and symptoms will suggest the different parts of the CNS that are being affected. The "time" criterion means that lesions (or symptoms) occur at different time points. So a person with two relapses a year apart would satisfy this criterion.

The main effects of the McDonald criteria were to improve the accuracy of diagnosis, and to enable MS to be diagnosed earlier. Two sets of modifications were made in 2005 and 2010.[2,3] The main effect of the 2010 revision was to simplify the criteria used to diagnose MS in someone with "pre-MS", known as clinically isolated syndrome (i.e. a single demyelinating attack). This meant that some people with CIS could be diagnosed as actually having MS after only one MRI. As we'll see below, this has had a major impact on how we interpret studies looking at the long-term outcome of people with MS.

As a result of these discussions and revisions, MS is now diagnosed if a person has had at least two separate flare-ups (the "time" requirement) affecting different parts of the brain (the "space" requirement). An MS relapse (also called an attack or an exacerbation) is defined as neurological symptoms that indicate demyelination; these symptoms must persist for at least a day (some say two days), and are not caused by fever or infection (which can worsen symptoms but are not associated with an inflammatory episode in the brain). The two flare-ups can be a current relapse (confirmed by a neurological exam or an MRI) and a prior episode that the person recalls. So for example, if a person has symptoms of tingling and numbness and recalls an episode of optic neuritis six months ago (i.e. sensory symptoms and optic neuritis indicate two different parts of the CNS are affected), that would meet the criteria for an MS diagnosis. If a person had two episodes of optic neuritis, this would not satisfy the criteria because only one part of the CNS (the optic nerve) is affected. Further evidence would be needed, such as an MRI showing multiple lesions affecting different parts of the brain. So this person would be said to have CIS until the "space" criterion was met.

As part of the effort to diagnose earlier, a new concept has emerged called radiologically isolated syndrome (RIS).[4] What this means is that a person with no MS symptoms happens to have a brain MRI and the scan shows some abnormalities that are MS-like. This may represent the very earliest signs of MS, although it isn't clear what proportion of people with RIS will ultimately develop MS, nor has it been determined if these people would benefit from an MS treatment.

Is CIS actually MS?

CLINICALLY ISOLATED SYNDROME (CIS) – or a single neurological attack (e.g. optic neuritis) –first attracted attention in the early 1990s when it was found that a majority of people with CIS subsequently developed MS if they also had an abnormal MRI.[5] This is in contrast to people with CIS with a normal MRI, for whom the risk of developing MS is very low (3% over a five-year period); at the 10-year mark, the 3% is about 11%, but is seemingly benign (i.e. no disability progression).[6]

CIS raised two interesting questions: Does it represent early MS, which could give researchers an idea of how demyelination progresses; and would treating CIS have more of an impact than treating MS? The latter question is the "stitch in time" idea that early treatment might prevent damage later on (presuming, of course, that CIS eventually becomes MS).

Whether or not CIS is essentially early-stage MS is still somewhat controversial. Taken on its own, a single neurological symptom suggestive of MS is actually MS in only a minority of cases. This is because people can have a wide range of symptoms, some of which indicate a medical condition (such as migraine), and some of which are for no reason at all (even healthy people have abnormalities on their MRI).

One example of this is optic neuritis, a common early symptom of MS that's experienced as vision problems (e.g. double vision, "jumpy" vision, blurriness, etc). In the Optic Neuritis Treatment Trial, only 1 in 4 people with optic neuritis and no other neurological symptom ultimately developed MS over the next 15 years.[7] Even a condition that resembles MS, such as transverse myelitis (an inflammation of the spinal cord), isn't a sure bet: an Australian study found that among people with transverse myelitis and no other signs/symptoms of MS, none developed MS over the next 2-3 years.[8] Other studies have found that among people with low-risk CIS, only about one-third go on to develop MS over the next few years.[9]

So a single attack of neurological symptoms isn't sufficient in itself for a diagnosis of MS because many other conditions can cause these symptoms. But the picture changes if the MRI is abnormal. If an MRI of the brain and spinal cord detects lesions that resemble MS lesions, it's much more likely that the CIS is really MS. Even one lesion is enough to increase the likelihood of having MS;[10] more lesions increase the likelihood further still. So MRI results are an important indicator of the risk a person has of developing MS.

There are numerous "red flags" that may crop up during an office visit that may indicate to your neurologist that it's unlikely you have MS. Your doctor will look at the whole picture: who you are, what is your medical history, what are your symptoms, and so on. If you're older (past 50 years), your CIS symptoms are less likely to be MS. If you have another illness that could explain your symptoms, MS may be ruled out. A variety of symptoms, such as headaches, seizures, nerve pain in your hands or feet, muscle spasms while asleep, and so on may suggest something other than MS.[11] Diagnosing MS is a difficult business, which is why a CIS/MS diagnosis is best made by an experienced neurologist.

There are also signs that indicate that MS is more likely. As mentioned above, more disease activity on an MRI (as indicated by the number and type of lesions) increases the likelihood that CIS will become MS. Earlier studies found that people with lesions on a baseline MRI and new lesions on a follow-up scan 3-6 months later were more likely to develop MS.[12]

From a person's point of view, more symptoms or more severe symptoms would intuitively seem to be a bad sign. But in a neurological exam, the number of different symptoms is significant only if it indicates that there is more than one lesion causing problems in different parts of the brain. So for example, if you are having vision problems and bladder symptoms, then there is more than one lesion. This is called multifocal (as opposed to monofocal) disease,[13] and denotes more widespread disease activity. But multifocal shouldn't be confused with multiple symptoms. A monofocal (i.e. attributable to one lesion) onset may result in more than one type of symptom. So make sure that your neurologist clearly explains what your symptoms mean.

When predicting who is at higher risk of developing MS, the specific symptoms are less important than what they represent in terms of how extensive is the amount of inflammation and demyelination. A greater burden of disease, as shown by more lesions, larger lesions and/or a multifocal onset, is a stronger warning that MS will develop.[14] Older people with CIS appear to have a lower risk of developing MS than younger people.[15] This may be because older people are less likely to develop new inflammatory CNS lesions,[16,17] or may indicate that they have somewhat better repair mechanisms since CIS was so late in developing.

African-Americans with CIS have a higher risk of developing MS than whites with CIS, which is likely due in part to genetic factors.[15] Women appear to have a two-fold higher risk of developing CIS than men, and a slightly higher risk of progressing to MS thereafter.[18]

Can CIS be treated?

CIS WITH MRI CHANGES SUGGESTIVE OF MS will develop into MS in most cases, although this may take several years. So the conventional wisdom is that early treatment – the earlier the better – will produce greater long-term benefits. Indeed, pharmaceutical companies were the early champions of CIS, no doubt hoping that medications would be more effective earlier in the course of the disease (with the added benefit of expanding the market for their products).

Over the past decade, there have been five landmark studies that have looked at the advantages of early treatment of CIS (a sixth study is included in the chapter on Aubagio). The first was called CHAMPS (for Controlled High-Risk Subjects Avonex Multiple Sclerosis Prevention Study) and included people with a single demyelinating neurological event (such as optic neuritis or transverse myelitis) as well as two or more lesions on their MRI.[19] In other words, these people were at high risk of developing MS. Everyone received a course of steroids and Tylenol (acetaminophen) for a couple of weeks, then one-half of the subjects received Avonex at the usual dose of one injection per week (the other half got a placebo injection). After three years, one-third of the Avonex group had developed MS compared to 50% in the placebo group. This was calculated to mean that treatment reduced a person's risk of "converting" to MS by 44%.

"Conversion" to MS is the term that's usually used, but it's a bit of a misnomer because if CIS actually is MS, then no conversion is needed. Rather, what it means is that fewer people taking Avonex met the criteria for an MS diagnosis. If they are diagnosed with MS later on, of course they had MS all along. So the conversion is better seen as a reclassification. As mentioned previously, the revisions to the diagnostic criteria have enabled more people with CIS to be categorized as having MS. So the "conversion" rate in CHAMPS would have been much higher (for both the treatment and placebo groups) if the study had been done after the revised diagnostic criteria came into effect.

Be that as it may, the results of the CHAMPS study earned Avonex a new indication as a treatment for CIS, and it wasn't long before other studies were launched to test competing products. The first was arch-rival Rebif, which is essentially the same drug as Avonex but taken on a more frequent schedule (and injected under the skin rather than in the muscle). A curious feature of the ETOMS (Early Treatment of MS) study was that it dosed Rebif as if it were Avonex (a low dose [22 micrograms] once a week) instead of being Rebif. This was a serious flaw of the study and the results were predictably poor. About 34% on Rebif developed MS within two years (CHAMPS was a three-year study) compared to 45% with placebo.[20] This wasn't deemed to be enough of a difference, so Rebif was not approved for the treatment of CIS in many countries. It would take over a decade for the usual dose of Rebif (44 mcg three times a week) to be tested in another CIS trial called REFLEX (REbif FLEXible dosing in early MS).[21] This time the results were somewhat better: after two years: 62.5% in the high-dose Rebif group developed MS compared to 85.8% in the placebo group (and 75.5% in a group receiving Rebif once a week). (More people in this study developed MS because they were using the new diagnostic criteria.)

The next study was BENEFIT (for Betaferon/Betaseron in Newly Emerging Multiple Sclerosis for Initial Treatment), which examined Betaseron (called Betaferon in some countries) compared to a placebo in 468 people with CIS.[22] In contrast to the ETOMS study, the trial investigators were clever enough to use the usual dose of Betaseron. At two years, 28% in the Betaseron group had developed MS compared to 45% in the placebo group (69% and 85%, respectively, using the new diagnostic criteria).

These results are remarkably consistent. About 45-50% of people in these trials developed MS over the next 2-3 years if they received no treatment. That risk was reduced roughly 30-40% if they started treatment with an interferon.

The late-comer to CIS trials was Copaxone, but when the results of the PRECISE trial were finally published in 2009 they were very similar.[23] Treatment reduced the risk of developing MS by about 40%.[24] Or to put it more precisely, treatment reduced the likelihood of people meeting the criteria for a diagnosis of MS.

What have we learned from CIS treatment studies?

THE CIS STUDIES INDICATE that if people at high risk of developing MS start treatment earlier, about one-third won't be diagnosed with MS over the next 2-3 years. So taken at face value, it would seem that early treatment can "prevent" MS (or at least delay an MS diagnosis). However, CIS trials leave us with several problems of interpretation.

The first is that if CIS were routinely treated, many people would receive a medication who might not need it. For example, in the CHAMPS trial of Avonex,[19] fully 50% of people taking a placebo for three years didn't develop MS. In fact, when this placebo group was started on Avonex, 50% still hadn't developed MS two years later.[25] So it could be argued that many people will do just fine for several years even without treatment, avoiding the need for regular injections and without incurring the substantial costs of the medication.

But it's important to realize that delaying a diagnosis of MS isn't the same as delaying the development of MS. Calling something CIS rather than MS is about the cut-off value of the signs and symptoms needed for an MS diagnosis – it isn't about whether or not the disease is present. The revised diagnostic criteria illustrated this when they allowed more people to be categorized as MS rather than CIS. As mentioned before, in the BENEFIT trial of Betaseron, when the new criteria were used, far more people "converted" to MS during the two years of that study.[22] With the old criteria, 45% in the placebo group were diagnosed with MS (and 55% were not); with the new criteria, 85% developed MS (and 15% did not). Keep in mind that these are the same people. The same was seen in the CIS trial of Copaxone: a 36% conversion rate using the old criteria and a 57% rate with the new criteria.[26] Again, this was the same group of people. In a practical sense what this means is that people with CIS are roughly 40-50% more likely to be diagnosed with MS today than if they went to see their doctor 10 years ago. It remains to be seen if these people with "new MS" (formerly known as CIS) will have the same outcomes over the long term as people with old-school MS.

An immediate consequence of a more permissive definition of MS is that it makes it more difficult to compare new and old studies of MS medications (since many of the people in the older CIS trials would now be considered to have MS). So it's difficult to compare an older CIS study (such as CHAMPS) with a new CIS study (such as the TOPIC trial of Aubagio) because the populations being studied are very different. This problem also affects MS trials since many people in an MS study today would not have been eligible a few years ago because they would have been diagnosed with CIS, not MS. What this means is that people enrolled in MS trials today are less severely ill than those entering trials two decades ago. (This is one of the reasons why in clinical trials today, the relapse rate is actually lower in people taking a placebo than the relapse rate in people on active medication in the old MS trials.)

Of course the incentive for making an MS diagnosis earlier is to start treatment earlier. But an earlier diagnosis may be a mixed blessing. It may be a relief to some that their puzzling symptoms now have a name, but it also means you have to come to terms with the label of MS and whatever that may entail. Uncertainty is hard; certainty can be harder when it comes to talking to your partner, children, employer and insurers.

An earlier diagnosis would certainly be worthwhile if starting a disease-modifying therapy sooner actually modified the course of the disease. But here we face two difficulties. The first is about whether the "new MS" (formerly CIS) is really MS. In other words, does it behave in the same way as MS? One way of looking at this is with natural history studies. These typically look back at people in MS databases to see how they did over the longer term – a researcher's way of skipping to the end of the book to see how things turned out. MS databases have been in place for decades and for most of that time there were no treatments available, so you can get a good snapshot of how a population of people with untreated MS will fare over time. We'll look at what these natural history studies have shown for MS in the next chapter. But right now we'll consider what they tell us about CIS.

The first impression you can get is that MS is becoming a more benign disease – that people can often have MS longer before they develop any disabilities. For example, if we assume it takes 25 years on average for someone to need a cane (EDSS 6), that same point may now be reached in 30 years. But this doesn't mean that MS is less aggressive – what's happening is a "frame shift". If you start counting out the 25 years from Time 0, if a person is now diagnosed five years earlier (i.e. at Time -5), then the 30 years for the person with the earlier diagnosis is the same as the 25 years for the person with the later diagnosis.

The way you categorize things can create wrong impressions. This has been called the "Will Rogers phenomenon", named after the American humourist for his famous remark ("When the Okies left Oklahoma and moved to California, they raised the average intelligence level in both states.") A shift in categories can create the illusion of change. This can be demonstrated with two groups of numbers: 1, 2, 3 and 4, 5, 6. The average for the first group is 2 (1 + 2 + 3 divided by 3), and for the second group is 5 (4 + 5 + 6 divided by 3). Now if you reclassify CIS (the 3 in this example) and move it into the second group (the MS group), the average goes down for both groups: 1 + 2 divided by 2 = 1.5 (formerly 2); and for 3 + 4 + 5 + 6 divided by 4 = 4.5 (formerly 5). If these numbers represented disease severity, both the first group (CIS) and the second group (MS) appear to be doing better, although they're the same people.

The "Will Rogers" effect was shown in a study comparing how the use of different diagnostic criteria changes the impression of what's going on.[27] Using the old criteria, 11% of people with CIS had a moderate level of disability (EDSS score of 3) after seven years, while with the new criteria it was only 7%. For people with MS, 46% using the old criteria reached an EDSS score of 3 after seven years, but only 27% did when the new criteria were used. So people in both the CIS and MS groups appeared to be doing better. But of course the people hadn't changed, only the cutoff values. So any change couldn't be attributed to a difference in how their cases were managed or whether they were taking more effective treatments. The only difference was the category they'd been put in. So we'll need to keep this cautionary tale in mind when we turn our attention to natural history studies of MS in the next chapter.

Should I start treatment for my CIS?

WE'VE SEEN THAT TREATING CIS CAN DELAY being diagnosed with MS for a few years, although it is also the mixed blessing of starting treatment earlier. But delaying a diagnosis isn't really worthwhile in itself – it's just forestalling the inevitable (in a majority of cases). So the real question is whether early treatment – the stitch in time – saves anything?

Overall, about 1 in 3 people with CIS will have little or no disability over the next 20 years,[28] so you wouldn't expect them to get much apparent benefit from treatment. On the other hand, about 50% will develop disabilities and early treatment might help in those cases. Determining who will have an easier time of it and who will develop disability is the tricky part. Unfortunately, from the outset of CIS, there's no way of predicting how someone will do over the longer term.

While intuitively it makes sense to fight a disease in its earliest stages, there is little objective data to support that decision, at least with the earlier crop of therapies. The CIS trials of injectable drugs showed that early treatment reduced the likelihood of being diagnosed with MS over the next 2-3 years. But in reality, all this means is that treatment delayed the next relapse – the one that's needed to meet the criteria for a diagnosis of MS. So this finding isn't surprising. All of the treatment trials show that MS drugs reduce the risk of relapse.

But two of those studies – BENEFIT (which looked at Betaseron) and CHAMPS (which looked at Avonex) – now have long-term data that can tell us more.

In the case of BENEFIT, once the original two-year study ended, people in the Betaseron arm were able to continue on treatment, and people on placebo were switched over to Betaseron.[29] So this allowed the researchers to look at the advantages of earlier treatment since the people originally assigned to Betaseron started treatment two years before people in the placebo group. The average number of relapses per year (called the annualized relapse rate) was lower in the people who started treatment earlier, but this was true only in the first year of treatment (when the delayed group was on placebo). The delayed-treatment people caught up with respect to relapse frequency as soon as they started treatment.

The most important area they looked at was progression of disability, as measured by a worsening EDSS score. But here they found no difference. A comparable number of people in both groups (about 1 in 4) showed progression after five years. In addition, a comparable number of people in both groups developed secondary-progressive MS (about 2%) over that same five-year period. Overall, there were some modest benefits with earlier treatment but these have to be weighed against the time, trouble and expense of self-injections for an extra two years.

The CHAMPS study of Avonex also followed-up people after the original three-year trial was completed. For this extension study, called CHAMPIONS (for Controlled High-Risk Avonex Multiple Sclerosis Prevention Study in Ongoing Neurological Surveillance), everyone received Avonex. So the original treatment group got a three-year head-start on the placebo group. The results differed slightly from BENEFIT but were essentially the same. Over the course of 10 years, people who had received immediate treatment had a lower annualized relapse rate in years 5-10 than those receiving delayed treatment. The delayed-treatment group never caught up with respect to their relapse rate – they continued to have more relapses over the next decade. However, there was no difference between the two groups with respect to MRI activity or disability. Ten years after being diagnosed with CIS, only 9% had reached an EDSS score of 4 (able to walk unaided for 500 meters). So earlier treatment didn't appear to provide much in the way of real benefits (other than fewer relapses). Part of the challenge of showing a treatment benefit was the low rate of disability overall. But then if there's a low risk of disability, this isn't a strong argument for starting a medication that you hope will prevent disability.

This doesn't necessarily mean that starting treatment as early as possible won't do some good. It isn't known if treatments have subtle effects on the disease process. One area that may benefit is cognition (your ability to think, remember and plan). A number of studies have shown that many people with CIS experience cognitive difficulties. The areas most affected are speed of processing information, memory and planning/problem-solving.[31-34] While this hasn't been a major focus of research, there was a suggestion of some cognitive improvement with treatment in the BENEFIT study.[35] This is an area that needs to be studied further.

The net result of all this research is that treating CIS will lower the risk of having a relapse, which in turn will delay being diagnosed with MS. However, there is little evidence to show that this short-term gain will translate to long-term benefits in delaying disability. There doesn't appear to be a big disadvantage to putting off the decision to start treatment for a couple of years.

Of course this only applies to the interferon drugs (the long-term follow-up of the Copaxone CIS trial isn't available yet). It may well be that starting treatment earlier with a more potent medication may be a better stitch in time for preventing disability. Among the newer drugs, only Aubagio has been studied in CIS.[36] The TOPIC trial showed that Aubagio lowered the risk of developing MS by 37-43% – very similar to what was seen in CIS studies of the interferons and Copaxone. No long-term data are available. More potent medications, such as Tysabri, Gilenya, Tecfidera or Lemtrada, haven't been studied in CIS, so it isn't known if they would have a greater impact if taken as early as possible in the disease course.

CHAPTER 3

WHAT CAN I EXPECT?

MS IS A DISEASE OF UNCERTAINTY. You never know how you'll feel when you wake up in the morning, when you'll have a relapse, or if the slow creep of the disease will steal away your ability to do the things you routinely do today. MS affects everyone differently – when they develop it, how their symptoms appear, and how quickly it progresses. This means that when you're first diagnosed, no one is able to predict what will happen in the years ahead.

There are some broad brushstrokes that can be applied. When MS is first diagnosed, about 85% will have the relapsing-remitting form of the disease (RRMS). This is characterized by periodic relapses (also called attacks or exacerbations), with full or near-complete recovery from the attack when the symptoms go into remission. You may then go for years without acute symptoms, which can give the mistaken impression that the disease is lying dormant. At some point, most people develop a secondary-progressive form (SPMS), in which relapses typically become less frequent but recovery from a relapse is poorer and there is a steady accumulation of disability. The third type is primary-progressive (PPMS), in which there is disability progression from the outset. A subgroup of people with PPMS may be categorized as progressive-relapsing MS, although it doesn't appear that progressive disease with relapses behaves any differently than PPMS without relapses.[1]

We can see from this scheme that the classification of MS is based on clinical observation – the pattern of relapses, and how quickly disability develops – rather than on the underlying disease process. This is reflected in the most recent description of MS, which largely categorizes MS according to inflammatory activity and whether or not disability is progressing.[2] True relapses are typically the result of inflammation in the CNS. This distinguishes them from false relapses (called "pseudorelapses"), which may feel the same but aren't caused by a flare-up in the brain. A pseudorelapse is when you feel your symptoms worsen temporarily when you become overheated (such as after exercise or a hot bath) or are running a fever (which neurologists call Uhthoff's phenomenon).

Relapses can cause temporary impairments, such as persistent numbness or difficulty walking, but these don't necessarily indicate disease progression. Many people will regain their function, although this may take several weeks or months (or years in some cases). In contrast, worsening disability is the result of degeneration of the nerve fibres in the brain and spinal cord. These two processes – inflammation and neurodegeneration – are linked but the precise nature of their relationship isn't entirely clear. We'll examine this later when we look at some of the warning signs of a more difficult course.

What can we learn from natural history studies?

IT'S VERY DIFFICULT TO GET A CLEAR PICTURE of how MS behaves if you look at individuals because the signs and symptoms vary so much from one person to another. This is likely due to slight genetic variations, the person's immune biography, different levels of exposure to environmental factors and how well people heal. These differences can be smoothed out by examining populations of people, with the broader view of providing less individual detail but a better overall perspective. These examinations can be done with population databases such as national patient registries or insurance databases, as well as with medical records from MS clinics.

One of the oldest MS databases is in Lyon, France, which has patient records dating back to 1957. For the first four decades, these people didn't have access to the current crop of MS drugs so this database provides a snapshot of what happens to untreated people with MS during their lifetimes. This is a true natural history study, showing the nature (behaviour) of a disease in the absence of treatment. The Lyon cohort was also the starting point for the European database for MS (called EDMUS) that was launched two decades ago.[3] Many of our ideas about the nature of MS got their start in Lyon.

The Lyon database includes information on 1,844 people with MS.[4] One of the goals the researchers had in examining the database was to see how long it took from a diagnosis of RRMS or PPMS to the development of different levels of disability. The key milestones they looked at were EDSS 4, EDSS 6, and EDSS 7.

The EDSS (Expanded Disability Status Scale) is an assessment of the degree of MS disability, or neurological impairment.[5] The EDSS scale is rated from 0 (no impairment) to 10 (death). For the lower range of the scale (0-3.5), the score is determined by neurological signs and symptoms (rather than mobility problems). For example, if you had a slight tingling sensation but no other symptoms, your EDSS score would be 1.0. Minimal symptoms in two areas (e.g. tingling and muscle weakness) would be an EDSS score of 1.5. If there is any disability, that would be rated as EDSS 2 or higher.

An EDSS score of 4 represents some impairment in mobility but the person is able to walk without aid or rest for more than 500 metres (1,640 feet, or about a third of a mile). EDSS 6 means you need a cane or other support to walk 100 metres (328 feet, or about the length of a Canadian football field). EDSS 7 means a person is unable to walk even a short distance without resting so a wheelchair is generally needed.

For people with RRMS in the Lyon cohort, the median time from diagnosis to an EDSS score of 4 was 11.4 years. To reach an EDSS of 6, the median time was 23.1 years; and to reach EDSS 7, the median time was 33.1 years. "Median" means that one-half of the people were above this mark and one-half were below. Other studies, such as the analysis of people in the London, Ontario, database, have reported a similar median time frame – about 20 years – before reaching EDSS 6.[6]

So in evaluating the typical risk of developing SPMS (which corresponds roughly to EDSS 4), there's a 50-50 chance that this progressive phase will begin about 11 years after diagnosis. If you were diagnosed at age 30, this would mean that there's a 50-50 chance of developing SPMS by your early forties. By your fifties, most people will require a cane to get around (EDSS 6). By your sixties, there's a 50-50 chance that you'll need to use a wheelchair (EDSS 7).

But before we think of these projections as cast in stone, it's important to insert a few cautionary notes. These time points don't refer to specific individuals. They are averages obtained from a population as a whole, so they can't be used to pinpoint what lies in store for a given person. But they do indicate that against the metronome of relapses, there is a background noise of a ticking clock.

Secondly, the criteria used to diagnose MS were different from today's criteria for much of the time that the Lyon database has been accumulating information, MRIs were not available until the 1980s, and there were no effective treatments until the mid-1990s (so arguably doctors were slower to diagnose MS because there was little they could do about it). All of these factors can easily put off a diagnosis by a few years. This means that determining the true starting point is a bit of a problem. If MS were diagnosed five years earlier, perhaps we should add five years to these milestones: 16 years to EDSS 4, 28 years to EDSS 6, and 38 years to EDSS 7. In fact, a more contemporary study of people with MS in British Columbia did find that the median time to reach EDSS 6 was 28 years,[7] which may be due in part to earlier diagnosis.

Another important consideration is whether these same time points apply in people who are on treatment. We'll look at this more closely later on in this chapter.

These reservations aside, a couple of important ideas emerged from the Lyon analysis. For people with progressive disease from the outset (PPMS), disability milestones were reached much sooner – 7.1 years for EDSS 6, and 13.4 years for EDSS 7. But whether a person with PPMS had relapses or not didn't affect the rate that disability progressed. This suggests that for this form of the disease (or during this time frame of MS), neurodegeneration is proceeding more or less independently of inflammation because whether or not inflammation (relapses) is happening, degeneration is occurring at the same steady pace.

MS has been described as a two-stage disease.[8] During the first stage, inflammation (represented by relapses and MRI lesions) predominates. In the second stage, neurodegeneration (an accumulation of nerve damage represented by worsening EDSS scores) predominates. But in the case of PPMS, progressive nerve damage is evident from the start, which has prompted some to question whether PPMS and RRMS are actually different diseases.

While this question is still the subject of debate, the general thinking is that PPMS is not a different illness. RRMS, SPMS and PPMS are believed to be different points in time in the evolution of MS.

Inflammation and neurodegeneration are both present from the beginning – long before any symptoms appear. When MS actually begins isn't known, but this is a fairly common situation in medicine since symptoms have to be intrusive enough to prompt a person to see their doctor. For MS, it's believed that there are about ten inflammatory flare-ups in the brain for every relapse that a person experiences.[9] When the symptom threshold is reached, the person experiences a relapse (although they often don't go to their doctor right away). A relapse may become noticeable earlier if an inflammatory lesion affects an especially sensitive part of the brain; this is what neurologists call an "eloquent" lesion, because it speaks to us in the language of symptoms and forces us to pay attention. Additionally, some symptoms are more frightening, which may prompt people to go to their doctor sooner rather than later.

Subtle signs of neurodegeneration may be present from the beginning, but the brain has a remarkable ability to compensate for any damage being done – at least initially. The brain repairs itself between relapses as best it can and much of the problem can go away. But as the years go by, a key threshold is reached. Nerve damage accumulates and the resulting neurological symptoms don't improve. It isn't clear if this is because the body's repair mechanisms run out of steam, key components needed for repair (such as the oligodendrocytes that produce myelin) become depleted or stop working properly, secondary inflammation causes more widespread damage, or the brain can no longer compensate for the accumulated damage and impairments become more obvious. In any event, this is when SPMS begins. In this regard, SPMS is a retrospective diagnosis: it's made only after the fact when your doctor sees that disability is worsening even though no relapses are occurring.

Looked at in this way, you could say that RRMS is essentially SPMS but not enough time has passed.[10] As for PPMS, it's MS but the early relapsing-remitting stage of the disease is missing. So PPMS isn't a different disease. It's just a later stage of the same disease – but the person has skipped the early stages (or the early stages were not seen by a doctor). This explains in part why PPMS is usually diagnosed at a later age than RRMS. Disability progression does typically start at an earlier age than for RRMS, which may be because PPMS is more aggressive or there is an earlier failure of the body's repair mechanisms. Genetic factors influencing immune response and myelin repair likely play a role as well.

An important implication is that progression from the outset appears to be no different than later-stage progression. The underlying disease process is believed to be same. This was suggested by perhaps the most important observation made by the Lyon group. Once someone reached EDSS 4 – whether they initially had RRMS or PPMS – their rate of disability progression was the same thereafter. So EDSS 4 represents a threshold. After that point, it will take an average of about five or six years to reach EDSS 6, and about 12 years to reach EDSS 7. It didn't matter if someone had gotten there because of RRMS or PPMS. EDSS 4 was the signal that henceforth there would be a steady accumulation of disability. In other words, once this point of no return had been reached, the body "forgot" how it got there.[11]

EDSS 4 is the tipping point – the point at which the brain's ability to repair damage and compensate for lost nerve cells can no longer counterbalance the destructive effects of inflammation and neurodegeneration. At EDSS 4, whether a person continues to have relapses or not doesn't appear to matter. The rate of progression of disability will be the same with or without relapses.

So MS is characterized by an initial phase when focal inflammation (seen as lesions on an MRI) is most apparent, followed by a second phase when neurodegeneration is more prominent. It isn't clear if inflammation begins the process of neurodegeneration, or whether degeneration occurs separately. But the current thinking is that inflammation lights the fuse that starts the degenerative process. Since the main effect of current MS medications is to target inflammation, this means that it's very important to start treatment early to restrict the damaging effects of inflammation on the brain and get the most benefit from the drug. Thus far, the first-generation injectable medications appear to have little or no effect on long-term disability, but it isn't clear why. One possibility is that they aren't effective enough in suppressing inflammation. It remains to be seen if better control of inflammation with more potent second-generation drugs will work better in slowing down the process of neurodegeneration.

The window of opportunity for controlling MS is very narrow. If EDSS 4 is the benchmark, one might think that there's a breathing space of 10-15 years after the diagnosis. But it's likely that MS medications have a diminishing impact on the disease process. The general opinion is that the first 2-5 years after diagnosis is when you will get the most benefit from a treatment. In the first few years, MS is a smoldering fire, and the goal is to prevent the fire from spreading and causing more damage.

The Lyon study suggested that once a person reaches EDSS 4 there will be a gradual accumulation of disability. But a second natural history study in France found that this may be overly optimistic. The Rennes MS clinic in northwest France has been collecting patient data since 1976.[12] In this analysis, there was the same two-stage process of inflammation followed by neurodegeneration – but the tipping point was EDSS 3. People were typically diagnosed with RRMS in their late 20s, and reached EDSS 3 in their early 40s, with men reaching this point about a year or two earlier than women. EDSS 6 was reached about 10 years later. One implication is that the effects of MS are in part related to a person's age. And in fact this was seen. People with RRMS were diagnosed at a median age of 28 years, whereas people with PPMS were typically diagnosed at age 39. However, both groups reached EDSS 3 at age 42, and both groups reached EDSS 6 in their early fifties. This reinforces the idea that PPMS is RRMS but the initial relapsing phase is hidden. But once the neurodegenerative phase begins, it proceeds at the same pace along the same course.

Natural history studies use different terms to indicate their starting point. Some say that the clock starts at "clinical onset", others at "disease onset". But these are not quite the same, nor is either completely reflective of what is going on. "Clinical onset" refers to when someone has enough symptoms to prompt them to see a doctor. So it's partly about symptoms, partly about the person's stoicism or denial, and partly about the neurological signs that a doctor detects during the exam. But of course the symptoms and signs may have started many years before. "Disease onset" ideally would be when MS begins, but no one knows when that is. So this uncertainty about the starting point is a problem. When we say that the average person with RRMS has 20 years or so before they reach EDSS 6, this can include someone who is diagnosed when they are 28 years old but who may have had symptoms five years before.

Over the past few years, changes in the criteria used to diagnose MS and the availability of disease-modifying therapies have made these natural history studies a little out of date. People with MS are different now. Because there are treatments available, doctors are more motivated to diagnose MS earlier. People themselves are more aware of MS – think of how many movies and TV shows depict (often inaccurately) someone with MS – so they may report their symptoms to a doctor more quickly or do a Google search to try to figure out what's going on.

Overall, looking at the MS population as a whole (rather than individual people), we can say that most people – about 85% or so – will start to develop impairments that don't improve after the relapsing phase has run its course. This is the beginning of irreversible disability, and it typically starts about 20 years after diagnosis. Not everyone will reach this point. As many as one in seven people will have "benign MS",[13] a controversial term that describes people with RRMS who don't develop moderate or severe disability (i.e. worse than EDSS 3) after 15 or 20 years of living with the disease. Some people will reach a certain level of disability and then plateau for many years. Natural history studies blur the fact that everyone is different, and that a person's individual disease course is difficult to predict.

Are there signs that I'll have a more difficult time?

WHEN YOU ARE FIRST DIAGNOSED WITH MS, it would be very helpful to know how bad it will be. Will I be able to keep working? Will I need to change my habits and lifestyle? Will I be able to walk down the aisle at my daughter's wedding? Unfortunately, it's very difficult for anyone to predict how things will turn out. MS isn't like a cancer, where a doctor can look at the size, location and grade of the tumour and predict fairly accurately how long you'll live if you don't start treatment. Some people with MS have terrible symptoms at the beginning but develop little disability; others appear to be minimally affected but progress rapidly. An MRI may light up with brain inflammation, but this in itself may not provide much of an indication of how severe things will be.

This is because the outcome will depend in part on the disease, but also on how well your body can defend itself against the disease. This isn't to say that some people are stronger and some weaker, or that some are fighters and some are not. The body's defences against MS are beyond anyone's control. Following an episode of demyelination, the body works hard to repair the damage and restore normal nerve function. Sometimes this will be effective, sometimes it won't be. So this is one factor – relapse recovery – that will determine how well a person will do in the long run.

How MS affects the body is also important. We can imagine that the type or location of damage will have a greater or lesser impact, although this may not be immediately apparent. A cut on your scalp may bleed profusely but may not be life-threatening, whereas a similar cut elsewhere on your body may bleed less but could be fatal. So we need to look at the types of injury that occur in MS.

Numerous studies have looked at various indicators that might help in determining the prognosis (i.e. knowing beforehand) of someone at the time they're diagnosed. Overall, three inter-related factors emerge. They are the type and severity of relapses; the frequency of relapses; and a person's recovery from relapses (which appears to be influenced by a person's age, sex and ethnicity). So let's look at each of these things in turn.

AS A GENERAL RULE, symptoms that seem worse at the beginning are a good indication of the severity of MS. Among the worrisome symptoms are: muscle weakness or paralysis; spasticity (muscle spasms or stiffness); uncoordinated muscle movements (ataxia); bladder or bowel problems; tremors; and dizziness or vertigo.[14-16]

During the initial workup, a neurologist will assess eight functional systems to determine which part(s) of the brain is affected. These functional systems are motor (pyramidal) function, cerebellar, brainstem, sensory, bowel/bladder, visual, cerebral (mental), and other. The functional system involved can be deduced from the signs and symptoms, such as muscle spasticity, balance problems, and so on. What's important to this scheme is that it's a bad sign if more than one functional system is affected. So sensory symptoms alone (such as tingling) have a better prognosis than sensory symptoms plus muscle stiffness, or visual problems plus bowel/bladder problems plus poor muscle control. For this early assessment, the number of functional systems affected and the severity of the symptoms will be the sole determinants of a person's disability score for people with an EDSS less than 3.5 (minimal to moderate disability). Beyond this point, walking ability becomes increasingly important in determining a person's disability score.

So having several functional systems affected at the beginning is a worse sign than if only one system is affected:[15] it indicates multifocal disease,[16,17] i.e. lesions in multiple locations in the brain, meaning that CNS inflammation is more widespread.

As mentioned previously, a relapse is a warning flare that inflammation is going on in the brain but the actual amount of ongoing inflammation may be 10-fold greater. To put it another way, about 90% of inflammatory flare-ups don't break through to the level of producing symptoms. More inflammation potentially means more relapses – and a greater frequency of relapses at the beginning would certainly seem to be another bad sign (and will definitely affect a person's quality of life). But this prognostic factor is time-limited: after the first couple of years, relapse frequency is no longer a good indicator of how well you will do.

Relapses are the most obvious symptom of MS, and this measure has traditionally been the benchmark to assess the effectiveness of medications in clinical trials. But as a prognostic factor, relapses say remarkably little about the future course of MS and there are several reasons for this. First, what is a relapse? The definition has changed over time and there is still a debate about whether symptoms that last 24 hours are too easily confused with temporary worsening or "false" relapses (clinical trials often require that symptoms last a minimum of 48 hours). Moreover, relapse frequency is largely determined by how often a doctor asks or how many a person reports. If you see your neurologist every three months, your relapse rate will be higher than if you see your doctor annually – a year after the event, many people forget about their relapses. One study that looked at this found that the relapse rate was more than twice as high if people saw their doctor every three weeks instead of every three months.[18] If we imagine the ultimate Don't Ask/Don't Tell scenario, the relapse rate will be close to zero – which will hardly represent how things are.

A further factor is that during the course of RRMS, the relapse frequency naturally declines over time. For example, one study found that relapses were more common among people in their 20s (on average about 1 relapse every 3 years), then steadily declined over the next few decades.[19] For each five-year period after diagnosis, the average relapse rate went down about 17% so that by the time a person was in their fifties, their relapse frequency was one-half of what it had been. This declining relapse rate was related to how MS behaves – most people in this study were not receiving an MS medication so what was seen wasn't a drug effect.

The study also showed some of the weaknesses of using relapses as a prognostic factor. Women had more relapses than men, and younger people had a higher relapse frequency than older people at diagnosis. But in both cases, the "lower risk" groups – men and older people – are known to have a somewhat worse long-term prognosis. They are, in fact, the higher risk groups. So clearly over the lifelong course of MS, relapse frequency as a prognostic factor loses its value.

A number of studies have indicated that relapse frequency in the first 2-5 years after diagnosis is important,[20,21] although this is somewhat controversial. Beyond that, relapse frequency probably doesn't have much impact on the development of disability. This is because the importance of inflammation, as represented by relapses, is superseded by neurodegeneration as MS progresses. It may be that once the inflammatory match has lit the tinder, the fire no longer needs a match to keep the flame burning.

Of course the frequency of relapses will be influenced by whether or not someone is on an MS medication. In this case, what appears to be important strictly speaking is not the frequency of relapses, but whether or not someone is responding to the drug (as shown by whether they're still having relapses). For example, a study of people on an interferon-beta drug found that their risk of disability progression was about 3-4 times higher if they had any relapses at all in the first two years of treatment.[22] A separate study, which looked at relapses and MRI for people during the first four years on an interferon, found that there was a 60% chance of disability progression if they had one or more relapses and as few as four new MRI lesions while taking the drug.[23]

The severity of a relapse can be offset to some degree by a person's recovery from it. Recovery reflects the state of the person's inbuilt repair mechanisms. These mechanisms cool down the inflammatory hotspot by re-regulating the immune response, re-growing the damaged myelin, removing the damaged bits and restoring function to the nerve fibre. This takes time, which is why relapse frequency – getting hit with more damage while you're in the middle of repair work – will influence your ability to recover.

Also important is functional recovery. If a damaged nerve can't regain its function, its signals can be shunted to adjoining nerve fibres so the message still gets through. If local damage is too extensive, these signals may get sent by another part of the brain. This adaptability ("plasticity") enables the brain to learn, and it allows the brain to compensate for some of the neurological problems it's having. It's the reason why low-level damage may not immediately register as a loss of function. The problem for many people with MS is that after many years of living with the disease, the repair work falls too far behind, the damage becomes too extensive, and the brain is no longer able to compensate.

THE SECOND FACTOR that predicts a more difficult time is early worsening of disease progression. But this idea needs to be clarified because when it comes to progression, there are actually two types that have to be distinguished. True progression is when the neurodegenerative phase is underway and there is ongoing accumulation of disability, as shown by a slowly worsening score on the EDSS scale. This requires a series of observations over a very long time period. If you are currently EDSS 5 (able to walk about 200 meters), and remember that you were able to walk unimpeded a few years ago, this probably represents true progression.

Researchers don't do clinical trials that run for 15 or 20 years. So in the context of a short-term drug trial, they'll often talk about "sustained disability progression". What this means is that a person's EDSS score worsens, and it hasn't improved by the time the doctor sees them again. The time between visits is typically three, six or twelve months. Of course in the long-term course of MS, this "EDSS progression" is only a snapshot. And EDSS progression may be misleading. Many people will have worsening disability during a relapse. In fact, it's not uncommon to lose one or two EDSS points overnight. For example, someone with mild sensory symptoms (EDSS

1) may find that these worsen during a relapse to a loss of touch sensation as well as a few new symptoms, such as slight changes in vision, a bit of clumsiness and slight muscle weakness. This would be enough to be re-scored as EDSS 3. But as these symptoms get better, the EDSS score drops back to 1 within a couple of months. So in the short term, there has been a two-point worsening; in the longer term, there is no net effect on function. So the "EDSS progression" has not resulted in true disease progression. And indeed, most people fully recover within two months, and even some subtle improvements can be detected up a year after a relapse.[24] So "EDSS progression" is better characterized as "worsening" to distinguish it from true progression.[25]

However, some people will have a relapse and they won't regain all of their function, at least in the short term. The risk of this happening is about 40-50%.[26,27] That is, a few studies have found that up to 40-50% of people experience a loss of 0.5 EDSS points during a relapse which isn't re-gained when the relapse quietens down, although this may be an overestimate since some people may improve over the next several months. A half-point isn't much and you might not notice it in your daily life. However, about 25% of people will experience more significant worsening – 1 or 2 EDSS points – following a relapse. This risk of losing some function following a relapse isn't the same for everyone. A person's age is one factor that will affect recovery – the younger you are, the more able you are to regain what was lost. About 90% of younger people with MS will make a full recovery from a given relapse, but this declines to about 70% in older people.[28]

An incomplete recovery from a relapse may mean several things. It can indicate that the attack was severe, causing too much damage to be fully repaired.[29] This severity may itself be a reflection of genetics – either the genetics of the immune response which determines the nature and extent of the attack; or the genetic mechanisms underlying the person's repair mechanisms, with some people healing better than others for reasons that aren't well understood.[30] So for example, men with RRMS will generally progress a bit faster, reaching EDSS scores of 3 (mild disability) or 6 (requiring walking assistance) about a year or two earlier than women.[12,31] People of African ancestry are generally held to be less likely to develop MS (although this notion has been challenged recently). If they do get MS, their symptoms are often more severe, recovery is poorer and they have a higher risk of developing SPMS, which is likely due to small but important differences in their genetics compared to whites of European ancestry.[32-34]

An incomplete recovery also leaves you vulnerable to additional attacks,[35] which may reflect that inflammatory activity hasn't fully died down or that neurons under repair are more susceptible to damage. This may explain why an important factor in estimating the risk of progression is the amount of time between relapses.[36]

The point of this discussion is not to belabour the fact that some people have a higher risk from the outset of developing progressive MS. But there are warning signs that deserve our attention. If your RRMS starts off with a lot of symptoms or especially severe symptoms, if you're having frequent relapses that don't give your body time to heal itself, and/or you don't fully recover from relapses, it would certainly indicate that your situation is more urgent – that you need to start treating the disease as soon as possible with the most effective medication.

Can treatment change the course of MS?

THUS FAR WE'VE LOOKED AT NATURAL HISTORY STUDIES of RRMS to examine what the course of MS looks like in people before treatments were available. The big question is: does treatment make a difference? Or to rephrase this slightly: Do the disease-modifying therapies (DMTs) actually modify the disease? This is the all-important question that must be asked before we turn our attention in the next section to the various pros and cons of the individual drugs.

The most scientific approach to this question would be to take two groups of people, one treated and the other untreated, and see how they do over the course of their lives. But this would mean that one-half of the participants would never receive treatment for their MS, which wouldn't be ethical. (Questions have been raised about the ethics of having a placebo group for even a two-year study.)

Another approach would be to look at people from the original treatment trials since they typically continue on therapy for years (if not decades) after the original trial has been completed. In such cases, the placebo group starts taking the drug during the extension phase. Unfortunately, such long-term studies tell us little or nothing about the effectiveness of a drug (despite their many claims).[37] Many people get tired of being in a trial and drop out. Once one-third of the participants are no longer in the trial, you can no longer pretend to come to any conclusions about the drug's effectiveness. Too much data is missing. One example is the long-term PRISMS study of Rebif, in which less than 60% of people in the original treatment groups completed six years on Rebif.[38] There was a similar problem with the Betaseron pivotal study: only 44% of the initial treatment groups started the fifth year on therapy (and only five people completed the study).[39] As a result, it couldn't be shown that Betaseron had a significant effect on relapses in the last three years of the study.

Many of these people in the Betaseron trial did continue treatment – either Betaseron or something else – outside the rigors of the clinical trial. About 88% of the original group were tracked down for a check-up at the 16-year mark, although detailed information was available for only 70% (including seven who had died).[40] Delaying the start of treatment for a few years appeared to have no impact on long-term outcomes. Some mathematical modelling showed that people with greater drug exposure did better than those with lower drug exposure.[41] But a person's outcome depended more on their disease characteristics before they started treatment rather than on the treatment itself.[42]

Similar problems were seen in the 15-year follow-up study of Copaxone (although the average time on drug was actually only 8-9 years).[43] The study found that people who stayed on treatment had very infrequent relapses, about one-half had minimal change in their EDSS score, and about two-thirds had not progressed to SPMS. However, we need to interpret these findings with caution. Generally speaking, people who were doing well on Copaxone continued in the study, while those who weren't doing well dropped out. So really this study is evaluating a very selective (and self-selected) group. They may have been "super-responders" to Copaxone; or, more troublingly, they may have been "super healers" who would have done just as well with no treatment.

So this type of long-term drug study isn't very helpful and may lead to the wrong conclusions. A different way of examining the question of long-term drug benefits is to troll through patient databases and compare outcomes in people with and without treatment. One such analysis was conducted in Italy and compared about 1,100 people taking an interferon-beta drug with about 400 people who received no treatment.[44] Those on treatment took longer to reach key disability milestones (EDSS 4 or 6), and developed SPMS later. These gains were a bit modest – treated people began the secondary-progressive phase about 3-4 years later than untreated people – but not insubstantial.

The Italian researchers also did two other analyses that were interesting. One looked at the benefit of taking an interferon for different lengths of time.[45] The overall risk of relapses and disability progression was substantially lower among those taking the interferon for more than four years compared to people on treatment for fewer than two years, so a sustained amount of time on therapy may be important. However, it's possible that the people who kept taking their treatment for four years did so because they were responding particularly well, which may have influenced the results.

Following on this, a separate analysis found that the best outcomes were seen in people who started treatment within a year of being diagnosed.[46]

These studies provide some measure of reassurance that treatments do have an impact, although the researchers themselves have not been especially enthusiastic cheerleaders.[47] But certainly the idea that treatment has a greater impact if taken early makes sense, and not just because of the idea of the "stitch in time". The MS drugs target inflammatory relapses. And as mentioned before, the impact of relapses on the long-term course of MS diminishes over time, so that 2-5 years after being diagnosed,[20,21] relapses are no longer a good predictor of how well a person will do over the long term. If relapses lose their importance, then we may make the inference that treatments that target those relapses will have a diminishing impact as well.

Other studies have tried to provide some hard numbers about the benefit of treatment. An analysis of all people treated with MS drugs in one Canadian province concluded that the long-term gain with treatment came out to about 0.1 EDSS point per year.[48] So over the course of 10 years, treatment would spare you about 1 EDSS point of disability. For those with mild disability this would hardly seem worthwhile. However, at higher levels of disability it can mean the difference between using a cane (EDSS 6) and needing a wheelchair (EDSS 7). We may wish the impact were more, but it isn't nothing.

Four of the more recent studies looking at the impact of treatment on disability arrived at different conclusions, a not uncommon situation in MS research. On the pessimistic side, a study in Brazil found that the amount of disability after 7-8 years was comparable in people on an MS medication and those receiving no treatment.[49] A retrospective study in British Columbia found that people taking an interferon didn't have a lower risk of disability compared to those on no medication, although the observation period was limited to five years.[50] There also appeared to be a bias in who was included in the study (i.e. more severely affected people were on drug, those with less severe disease were more likely not to start treatment), which probably underestimated the impact of treatment. On the more optimistic side, several studies – including two large studies in Italy and Sweden – have indicated that long-term treatment will delay the onset of secondary-progressive MS.[51,52]

In examining this question of the impact of treatment, a further complication is the general observation that people with MS enrolled in trials these days appear to progress more slowly than people did two decades ago.[53] Nowadays, it takes people longer to reach the stage of irreversible disability. We can speculate any number of reasons why this may be. For example, people are diagnosed earlier or start treatment sooner, which would support the benefits of early treatment. Or it may be that less severely affected people are entered into trials, whereas those with more severe symptoms skip trials and go on treatment immediately (i.e. a selection bias in clinical trials).

So determining the long-term impact of the interferon-beta drugs and Copaxone is challenging (and the other drugs haven't been in use long enough). What treatments do over the long-term course of MS would seem to be the most essential question to research, and yet it's extremely hard to investigate. In part this is because of the nature of MS itself – highly individual, highly variable, and with the main measure of disease (relapses) naturally declining over time whether treated or not. It's probably fair to assume that treatment will have the greatest impact if taken early – within a year or two of diagnosis – and if people keep to the regimen for at least five years. Maintaining this discipline may buy you time – perhaps several years without significant disability, and may delay the time when irreversible disability begins.

It's also important to keep in mind that against the uncertainty of the benefits of treatment are the certainties of the typical course of MS. Without treatment, most people with RRMS – about 85% or so – will progress to SPMS at some point. So every effort needs to be made to slow down progression as much as possible within the time available.

CHAPTER 4

IS PREGNANCY A "TREATMENT" FOR MS?

IT WASN'T VERY LONG AGO that doctors routinely told women with MS not to have children. This wrongheaded bit of advice has been completely reversed in recent years. It's now well-established that MS disease activity diminishes during pregnancy, with relapses generally returning only after the baby is born. This is believed to be due largely to the hormonal changes that occur during pregnancy and the effect of these hormones on the immune system.

From an immune standpoint, a developing fetus, with its antigens from the father, is a "foreign intruder".[1] "A stranger she/preserves a stranger's seed", as Aeschylus once wrote. So one of the changes that the mother's body must undergo during pregnancy is to lower the reactivity of the immune response so the body doesn't "reject" the fetus. In this regard, we can think of pregnancy as an "immune modulated state", not unlike the immune modulation that occurs while taking an MS medication.

So pregnancy acts in a similar way as an MS medication. Indeed, the near 80% reduction in relapses during the third trimester of pregnancy is greater than the relapse reduction seen with MS drugs. This has prompted some people to ask: is pregnancy a treatment for MS? And is it the most effective treatment of all?

What happens to MS during pregnancy?

RELAPSES TYPICALLY BECOME LESS FREQUENT during pregnancy, most notably in the third trimester (months 7-9), then increase again in the first three months after giving birth. In months 4-6 after childbirth, MS disease activity usually settles back to the same relapse rate as the person was experiencing in the year before becoming pregnant.

These observations were made in the Pregnancy in MS (PRIMS) study.[2] But while people have emphasized the risk of increased disease activity in the three months after childbirth, what's often overlooked is that 72% of women in the PRIMS study did not experience a relapse in the three months following childbirth. So while there is an increased risk of relapse after giving birth, most women won't experience a relapse – something to consider when you're deciding whether it's best to breastfeed or to re-start your MS therapy instead.

MS doesn't appear to have any major effects on the pregnancy itself. There's no evidence that women with MS will have a more difficult pregnancy, nor are they are more likely to have complications during pregnancy and childbirth.[3,4] There's little evidence that MS has any effect on the fetus.[4] You can also rest assured that MS doesn't increase the risk of a miscarriage, birth defects or having the baby born prematurely. Babies may have a slightly lower birth weight, but this doesn't appear to have any health consequences either during infancy or during the life of the child.[5,6]

If some women experience a surge in MS disease activity in the first few months after childbirth, it's fair to wonder if this has any long-term consequences. Will a pregnancy make your MS progress more rapidly?

This doesn't appear to be the case. Studies have shown that pregnancy doesn't influence the development of long-term disability.[7-9] A three-month spike in relapses is a small concern when considering the life-long course of MS.

Of course the question of whether pregnancy worsens MS is just one side of the coin, and researchers have since flipped this over. Instead of wondering if pregnancy may be harmful, was it possible that pregnancy was actually helpful? So instead of focusing on relapse activity after childbirth, they looked at whether the decrease in relapses during pregnancy was more important to the long-term course of MS. Maybe the hormonal changes in pregnancy did something to reset the immune response – making pregnancy in effect an MS treatment.

This thought occurred to one group of researchers twenty years ago. While working on a study about MS risk, they observed that women with three or more children tended to be less likely to develop MS than women with fewer children or none.[10] Unfortunately, almost two decades passed before this question was investigated in a more systematic way. The AusImmune study looked at women in Australia to see if their risk of developing CIS/MS was influenced by having had children.[11] The study found that for women with children, the risk of CIS (i.e. a first demyelinating event) was about 50% lower per child. (As you might expect, having children didn't affect a man's chances of developing CIS.)

If we compare these results to the CIS trials (see Chapter 2), then having one child was about as effective a "treatment" as Copaxone or one of the interferons. Having two children was much more effective than the injectable MS drugs. These results certainly suggested that pregnancies had a protective effect.

Preventing the development of MS isn't the same as actually treating it once it's established. So it's also important to ask: is there any evidence that having children has a long-term impact on relapses and progression?

One small study looked at relapses during and after a pregnancy.[12] Like others before it, it found that the overall frequency of relapses went down during pregnancy, then increased in the three months afterward. But when the researchers looked at what happened over the longer term, they found that the relapse frequency went down to less than one-half of what it had been before, and stayed low over the next six years. Part of this effect may be due to the declining relapse rate that's part of the normal course of MS. But there was a hint that pregnancy may have somehow reset or dampened the abnormal immune response and quietened down the MS.

Two studies then looked at the immune-modulating effects of pregnancy to see if there was a "treatment" benefit over the longer term. An initial study in the Netherlands found that a woman's pregnancies didn't seem to influence her risk of developing secondary-progressive MS (SPMS) for better or worse.[13] However, another group subsequently examined this issue in a different way by comparing the medical records of four groups of women with MS: those without any children, those who had children either before or after they were diagnosed with MS, and those who had children both before and after developing MS.[13] Looking over an 18-year time-frame, they found that women who'd had children at any time had a 39% lower risk of progressing to EDSS 6 (requiring a cane) compared to women with no children. The risk of progression was also slightly lower for women who'd had a child after being diagnosed with MS.[14] While this is only one study, a 39% reduction in disability progression would certainly be the envy of any of the MS therapies currently on the market.

Why does MS improve during pregnancy?

WHEN CONSIDERING THE QUESTION OF WHY MS improves during pregnancy then worsens in the first few months after childbirth, the most obvious thing to investigate is hormone levels. During pregnancy there's a surge in various hormone levels, most notably of progesterone and the estrogens estradiol (known as E2) and estriol (E3).

Progesterone and estriol seemed especially promising. Progesterone is a hormone that supports gestation or pregnancy (hence the name). Although it's not unique to pregnancy and levels fluctuate during menstruation, progesterone levels surge about 50-fold as the developing placenta takes over the job of producing the hormone. Estriol is not detectable in normal circumstances, but during pregnancy it represents about 90% of the estrogens produced.[15]

During pregnancy, progesterone modulates the immune response, reducing the inflammatory (Th1 and Th17) response and boosting the activity of regulatory T cells (Tregs), which lower the inflammatory (and autoimmune) response.[16-18] Progesterone may also promote remyelination of nerve fibres.[19]

One important role of Tregs is to promote immune tolerance so the mother's body doesn't reject the fetus. These shifts in immune function have their downside: immune modulation means that during pregnancy, women are more susceptible to certain infections and, conversely, if the mother has to fight off an infection during her pregnancy, this immune activation may put the developing fetus at risk.

As for the estrogens, a number of studies have suggested that estriol E3 boosts the anti-inflammatory (Th2) response, shifting immune cells to a less inflammatory profile.[15,20,21]

Estradiol E2 directly influences both the innate and adaptive immune systems,[22] and estradiol receptors can be found both on T and B cells.[23] Interestingly enough, low levels of estradiol appear to promote inflammation whereas high levels have an anti-inflammatory effect,[24,25] with one study reporting that higher levels of estradiol were associated with less disease severity.[26]

These findings led to a landmark study called POPART'MUS, which looked at whether hormone treatment immediately after childbirth (i.e. the postpartum period) could reduce the higher rate of relapses seen during that three-month period.[27] While the full results haven't been published, early results suggested that the study was a failure.[28] The relapse rate in the 12 weeks after giving birth was only marginally lower with hormone therapy compared to placebo (0.90 vs. 0.97). And there was no benefit on relapses in subsequent months as well.

This seemed to decide the issue and quashed some of the enthusiasm for using hormones as a treatment for MS. But in a real sense the question hadn't been addressed, and what POPART'MUS found had already been shown. Prior studies had already suggested that hormone therapy, in the form of oral contraceptives, had only a limited impact on the development of MS.[29,30] Conversely, other types of hormonal manipulation, such as the regimens used for in vitro fertilization (IVF), will actually worsen MS if the woman doesn't become pregnant after IVF.[31,32]

But a lack of effect on relapses with hormone therapy doesn't necessarily mean that hormones don't have an impact on the long-term disease course.

How could hormones alter the MS disease course?

THE PROFOUND INFLUENCE OF FEMALE HORMONES on immune function could have several important effects on MS progression. Estrogens have been shown to alter the T cell and B cell profile in people with RRMS or SPMS,[15] potentially making the immune response less damaging. But there are also "upstream" effects: pregnancy hormones actually regulate the genes that govern inflammation, although this retooling appears to subside by the third trimester of pregnancy.[33]

In addition, there are dozens of studies using the animal model of MS that have reported that estrogens can protect cells in the brain, such as neurons and oligodendrocytes (which make myelin).[34-37] A further suggestion is that progesterone can slow the passage of activated immune cells into the CNS,[38] and promotes the repair of damaged myelin.[18,39]

So a great deal of research supports the hypothesis that female hormones may have therapeutic effects. Unfortunately, only one small pilot study over a decade ago has investigated this possible MS treatment. The trial found that a once-daily dose of estriol (given as an 8-mg pill) in non-pregnant women substantially reduced the number and size of inflammatory lesions seen on the MRI.[40] There was also an improvement in cognition in women with RRMS, but not in those with SPMS. A phase II trial of estrogens/progesterone in Italy was announced in 2005 and should have been completed in 2009, but the study appears to be missing in inaction. A phase II study looking at estriol as an add-on to Copaxone has been in the works since 2007, but no results have been published. A third study of estriol add-on therapy to improve cognition was announced in 2011. The study is said to be recruiting people, but again there are no results.

Estriol is an attractive candidate for an MS therapy. Compared to the other two estrogens (estradiol and estrone), estriol is generally considered to be safer[41,42] (estradiol, because it stimulates cell proliferation, is associated with a risk of cancer). So estriol is commonly used as a hormone treatment in some countries for women going through menopause.[43-45] Long-term treatment with estriol does not appear to be associated with an increased risk of ovarian or endometrial cancer.[46] There are some studies that suggest that estriol may increase the risk of breast cancer,[47-49] so this will need to be investigated more thoroughly.

THE PROMISING RESULTS of hormone therapy in MS pose something of a conundrum. If female hormones are beneficial, why are women much more likely to develop MS? There have been numerous speculations but no firm answers. Some have suggested that women are more likely to inherit genes associated with MS susceptibility,[50] that having two X chromosomes increases the MS risk,[51] or that males have a lower risk because of their Y chromosome.[52]

Part of the higher MS risk may be attributable to the interaction of estrogens and vitamin D. While low vitamin D levels have been associated with a higher risk of MS, laboratory studies have suggested vitamin D supplements can reduce the severity of MS – but perhaps only in women.[53] Vitamin D appears to have more potent immune effects in women,[54] although it isn't clear why this would be.

Perhaps more important are the sex differences during the course of MS. Women may have a higher risk of developing MS, but men generally progress more rapidly and may have worse outcomes (although this notion has been challenged[55]). It may be that after developing MS, female hormones are able to reduce the damage caused by inflammation or are better able to promote neuronal repair.[20,56,57]

FEMALE HORMONES may become a useful add-on treatment taken in conjunction with an MS therapy, but is this an option for men? One side effect would be breast growth, which might not be well-received by men. But an alternative treatment may be the male hormone testosterone. Since males are less likely to develop MS, it was hypothesized that testosterone may have a protective effect. Castration studies (in animals) have shown that inflammation and demyelination worsen when testosterone is withdrawn.[58] In line with this was the finding that men with low testosterone appeared to have a five-fold higher risk of developing MS.[59]

A small pilot study tested the theory in 10 men with RRMS, who applied a testosterone gel (10 g containing 100 mg of testosterone) over a six-month period.[60] Muscle mass increased, as you might expect; cognitive function and brain volume also improved, as you might not expect. However, the treatment had no effect on the number or size of inflammatory lesions seen on MRI. A follow-up report from the same study found that testosterone increased the production of nerve growth factors in the brain,[61] so hormonal therapy may provide some measure of protection against neuronal injury. A Canadian phase II study plans to look at whether testosterone can reduce MS fatigue in men, but no results have been published yet.

Does breastfeeding improve MS?

BEFORE WE FINISH UP DISCUSSING the effect of hormones on MS, we should make a quick comment about breastfeeding. MS treatments and breastfeeding are generally either/or: either you re-start treatment soon after childbirth and forgo breastfeeding, or you breastfeed and remain off treatment until the baby is weaned. This is because of concerns about the drug passing from the mother's milk to the baby. As a result, many women are faced with the issue of whether it's better to breastfeed or to take their MS medication. There's no right or wrong answer to this question. It will be up to you to decide what's best for you and your baby.

With respect to the impact of breastfeeding on MS, it's possible that nursing your baby may protect against relapses because it delays the return of menstrual periods (called lactational amenorrhea); it has been suggested that this hormonal effect may lower the risk of a relapse. A small study in the U.S. found that women with MS who exclusively breastfed for at least two months were 5-7 times less likely to have a relapse after giving birth than women who didn't breastfeed.[62] However, the evidence is decidedly mixed. Some studies have found that exclusive breastfeeding has little impact on relapses.[63,64] It may be that women who breastfeed are simply healthier than those who choose not to breastfeed, so their chances of having a relapse are lower overall.[63]

Part II

UNDERSTANDING MS MEDICATIONS

CHAPTER 5

WHAT ARE THE INTERFERONS?

IN THE 1970S AND 1980s, researchers liked to debate the fundamental nature of MS: was it an autoimmune disorder, or was it caused by a virus (or both)? Interferons would become the first of the disease-modifying therapies for MS in large part because they could accommodate both of these stories.

The word "interferon" was coined in 1957 to describe a type of signalling protein (called a cytokine) produced by cells that "interferes" with viruses.[1] When a cell becomes infected with a virus it releases interferon, which acts as a signal flare to neighbouring cells. Some cells respond by shutting down production of their internal machinery and others will self-destruct, actions meant to limit the spread of the virus. Interferon also stimulates the immune response. Two important effects are to induce production of natural-killer cells, which are able to target and destroy infected cells; and to boost the ability of MHC (major histocompatibility complex) molecules to present viral proteins to immune cells such as T cells (discussed in Chapter 1).

Interferons became a focus of attention in the early 1980s for several reasons. There was a growing understanding of the complexities of the immune response; viral illnesses such as herpes (and human immunodeficiency virus [HIV] later that decade) were becoming more high-profile; and there was interest in the possible role of viruses in the development of cancer (such as human papillomavirus [HPV] and cervical cancer).

From the first, interferons seemed likely to be important in MS because of this connection both with viruses and with the immune response. Natural interferon levels were found to be elevated in the cerebrospinal fluid of people with MS,[2] suggesting that something – presumably a virus – was acting as a stimulus. Others noted that people with MS produced a lower amount of interferon in response to a viral infection,[3] indicating that the immune response was somehow impaired. In either case, it seemed reasonable that more interferon might do some good in MS.

If interferon were a chemical, it could be synthesized in a lab and mass produced like other drugs. However, it's a biological substance (like insulin), so it needs to be produced by cells or living organisms and the technology to mass-produce "biologicals" was largely lacking in the 1970s. It was only in the 1980s that genetic recombination techniques were sufficiently developed that large-scale production of biologicals became feasible. What genetic recombination involves is extracting a gene and inserting it into the genetic code of a rapidly dividing cell, co-opting that cell to make it a mini manufacturing plant that will pump out the biological product. In the case of Betaseron, a human interferon gene was transplanted to *Escherichia coli*, a species of bacteria that normally lives in the digestive tract. For Avonex and Rebif, a human interferon gene was inserted into a Chinese hamster ovary cell since reproductive cells divide more rapidly than other cells.

One challenge was that "interferon" actually designates a group of cytokines and there are many different types, which are named after Greek letters (alpha, beta, gamma). The first trial in MS in 1981 used interferon-beta, administering it in a series of injections into the spines of 10 people with MS.[4] A year later, five people showed some improvement – their relapse rate went from 1.8 relapses per year to 0.2 relapses per year (one person got worse). It wasn't clear why interferon seemed to improve relapses, so the researchers covered all bets by concluding that the results supported the notion that MS was caused either by a virus or by a dysfunctional immune response to viral infection. A subsequent report found that when the placebo group started receiving interferon injections, they too showed an improvement in their relapse rate.[5]

At the same time, a different type of interferon (the alpha form) was also reporting positive results in RRMS.[6] However, two larger studies subsequently found that many people with MS got worse when treated with interferon-alpha,[7,8] so this line of research was largely abandoned (although interferon-alpha is still used to treat other diseases such as melanoma). The same happened with interferon-gamma, which was shown to significantly worsen MS.[9]

That left interferon-beta. Fortunately, an early study found that injecting it under the skin was as effective as injecting into the spine,[10] so people were spared that particular misery. But it still needed to be injected, in part because proteins are digested by the powerful acids in the stomach if taken by mouth. (Oral formulations of interferon-alpha and -beta would later be tested but the results were not that impressive.[11,12])

These studies were the preamble: what followed in the 1990s was more promising, and more political. In 1993, the results of the first large phase III trial showed that interferon-beta significantly reduced the frequency of relapses in people with relapsing-remitting MS.[13] After two years, the overall relapse frequency was reduced about one-third (from 1.27 to 0.84 relapses per year) with the higher dose that was tested. Over the first four years, the reduction in relapses was slightly lower at 30%.[14] However, the drug appeared to have little or no effect on disability progression. Despite these rather modest benefits, interferon-beta did do something – and as such it represented a landmark in MS treatment. The drug, now called Betaseron (Betaferon in some countries), was approved by the U.S. Food and Drug Administration on July 23, 1993.

Betaseron was designated an "orphan drug" in accordance with the U.S. Orphan Drug Act of 1982, which grants certain privileges to manufacturers to encourage them to produce medicines for rare diseases. "Rare", according to this bill, means a disease that affects fewer than 200,000 people in the U.S., which required some pushing and shoving to get the number of Americans with MS to fit below that mark (the current estimate is over 400,000). As an orphan drug, Betaseron should have had seven years of market exclusivity without any competitors, but a second interferon was able to slip onto the market.

Avonex (interferon-beta-1a) is very similar to Betaseron (interferon-beta-1b) but it's administered as an injection into the muscle (rather than under the skin) and at a considerably lower dose. The dose and frequency of interferon injections have an important impact on the effectiveness of the drug, as later studies would show.[15,16] So Avonex had less of an effect on relapses and little impact on MRI measures of disease activity. Among those completing the pivotal study, the relapse rate was reduced about 18% – roughly half of the effect seen with Betaseron.[15] However, the study was designed quite cleverly to focus on disability. And on this measure, the trial was able to show that Avonex was more effective than placebo in slowing the progression of disability.[17] At two years, about one-third of people in the placebo group had sustained disability progression compared to 22% of those treated with Avonex. This sounds like quite an impressive difference, but people in the study had minimal disability and a follow-up study found that the "sustained disability" they were measuring wasn't very sustained: the EDSS score subsequently improved in many people taking the placebo.[18,19] So what was being measured was short-term impairments due to relapses rather than true disability. However, this claim – that Avonex had an effect on disability – would later appear in its label.

Since the Orphan Drug Act barred new interferons from the market once Betaseron had been approved, Avonex could only get approved if the FDA decided that it wasn't the same as Betaseron. It had to be a different drug. In normal circumstances this might be a problem since Avonex and Betaseron are essentially the same compound. But in the legal arena, different rules apply. Even if two drugs are the same in terms of their chemical properties, the FDA can rule that a drug is different if it's superior. "Superior" in this context means that it's more effective, or has a better safety profile.[20] Both of these criteria – effectiveness and safety – don't need to be met.

Showing that one drug is more effective than another is difficult, expensive and time-consuming: it usually means you have to do a head-to-head study comparing the two drugs. But the burden is less onerous if you want to make a safety claim. If you can show some safety advantage, the FDA may decide that your drug is superior (even if it's less effective or has other safety issues). Perhaps most importantly, a multimillion dollar head-to-head study isn't needed to make a safety claim.

Because of these rather arcane regulations, Avonex was able to get approved because of how it's injected. An injection deep into the muscle is less likely to cause severe skin damage (called necrosis) than an injection under the skin. This was enough for the FDA to designate that Avonex was superior, meaning that it was different enough to be marketed. So the FDA approved Avonex in May 1996; since it too was an orphan drug, it was granted market exclusivity for seven years.

This political maneuvering meant two things. There were now two interferons available to treat MS (along with the non-interferon, Copaxone). And the third interferon, Rebif (interferon-beta-1a), which is the same drug as Avonex, was left waiting in the wings. Rebif did its own phase III trial, called PRISMS[21] (for Prevention of Relapses and Disability in MS) – note the emphasis on disability in the title – which earned it approvals in various countries, but it wasn't able to be marketed in the U.S. It wasn't until 2002 that Rebif was able to break through this impasse by going head-to-head with Avonex.

Over the past decade, Rebif has thrown the dice a few times in comparative studies. The first of these was EVIDENCE, which pitted high-dose Rebif given three times per week versus once-weekly Avonex.[22] At the end of six months, 75% of people taking Rebif had experienced no relapses compared to 63% of those taking Avonex, sufficient for Rebif to claim that it was more effective than Avonex. (For the more usual way of reporting results, the relapse rate was 0.29 with Rebif and 0.39 with Avonex.) But this extra potency came at a cost: people taking Rebif were three times more likely to have skin reactions at the site of injection and were twelve times more likely to develop antibodies that could neutralize the effects of the drug. (The importance of these neutralizing antibodies would become a hotly-debated topic in the years to come.) A follow-up report found that Rebif was also better than Avonex in reducing inflammatory activity in the brain.[23]

These results were enough for the FDA to decide that Rebif and Avonex – although identical – were not the same.[20] There was no need to establish why one might be better than another, although it was generally assumed that the higher dose and the more frequent injections produced a better effect. So Rebif was finally allowed to be sold in the U.S. in 2002 – about a year before Avonex's exclusivity arrangement was set to expire. This meant that the ABC drugs (Avonex, Betaseron, Copaxone) had to make room for Rebif (with the four drugs commonly abbreviated as CRAB).

Are the interferons effective in other forms of MS?

IN THE SPACE OF A DECADE, people with MS went from having no effective drugs to treat their disease to having four – three interferons and Copaxone (discussed in the next chapter). All of the drugs were only modestly effective, reducing the frequency of relapses by about one-third for the MS population as a whole. Of course individual results, as the disclaimers are wont to say, will vary.

Having three interferons that were more or less the same created some unusual circumstances. There was the "float all boats" phenomenon: three companies promoting their own brand of interferon created a flood of noise that raised everyone's profile. At the same time, there was little brand differentiation in people's minds and doctors were remarkably uncommitted to recommending one treatment over another. Their general approach to patients was essentially: Here are the drug videos, take your pick. In effect, the message was that any treatment was better than nothing, but the specific therapy didn't matter since all had the same modest effect. This non-directive approach may have contributed to the problems doctors would have a decade later when some people, when asked for their preferred treatment, opted for surgery for chronic cerebrospinal venous insufficiency (CCSVI) rather than one of the injectables.

Of course there were differences among the interferons. The most obvious one was dosing. Betaseron was injected every other day, Rebif was three times per week and Avonex was once a week. Betaseron and Rebif were injected under the skin (subcutaneous), whereas Avonex was injected into the muscle (intramuscular). These were small differences, but many of the hundreds of interferon studies over the next decade fretted over them with jesuitical zeal. A great deal of attention was focused on three key questions: Do the interferons work in other types of MS? Is there a better dose? And is one drug superior to the others? To the more jaded, these questions might appear to be about market expansion, profit-taking and market share, respectively. But a great deal of information was nonetheless gleaned about the interferons in MS.

Regarding other types of MS, we've seen that all of the interferons are effective in clinically isolated syndrome (CIS) (Chapter 2). The three studies were the CHAMPS trial of Avonex, the BENEFIT trial of Betaseron, and the REFLEX study of Rebif.[24-26]

A more urgent need was to show that the interferons were effective in people with progressive forms of MS. This was a far more challenging proposition. In RRMS, interferons work primarily by reducing inflammation, as shown by their effect on relapses and inflammatory MRI lesions. However, once the secondary-progressive phase of the disease has begun, the development of disability is largely attributable to neurodegenerative changes rather than inflammation.

Unfortunately, there's little evidence that interferons have an effect on the neurodegeneration seen in progressive MS. But the hope was that these drugs, by reducing relapses in people who were still having relapses, might slow the process somewhat.

So three studies in turn looked at the impact of interferons in SPMS: the European Study Group trial of Betaseron, the SPECTRIMS trial of Rebif, and the IMPACT trial of Avonex. Betaseron was shown to delay progression by about a year.[27] In the follow-up report, fewer people worsened by two EDSS points after three years of treatment with Betaseron, although this benefit was primarily seen in those who were still having relapses.[28]

In contrast, Rebif was largely ineffective. The drug did reduce relapses in those people who were still having them and reduced brain inflammatory activity, but it had no impact on disability progression.[29,30] This probably indicates a difference in the people being studied rather than a difference between Betaseron and Rebif. In SPECTRIMS, people were a little older and most were no longer having relapses, whereas less than one-third of people in the Betaseron trial were no longer having relapses. Since interferons primarily affect relapses, there were fewer people in the Rebif trial likely to show an effect. In the IMPACT trial, Avonex had no effect on progression as it's usually assessed with the EDSS.[31] However, the investigators also used a second measurement scale (the MS Functional Composite, or MSFC), and here there was a difference, which was largely attributable to improvements in arm function and cognition.

So overall, these were not brilliant results, but they were sufficient for all three drugs to be used in people with relapsing forms of MS, which means both RRMS and relapsing SPMS. The practical result was that people could continue taking an interferon even if they were getting worse. But the more likely scenario was that people would stop taking their treatment if they weren't seeing a benefit. And clinicians weren't especially keen to press the point because of a general sense that interferons weren't effective in progressive MS. This impression was confirmed years later in an analysis of all SPMS trials, which concluded that the interferons don't prevent the development of disability.[32] There was a short-term gain in terms of reducing disability related to inflammation, but no longer term benefit.

Few studies have investigated interferons in primary-progressive MS. While one phase II study found that Betaseron had a small effect on MRI measures,[33] a systematic review concluded that there is little evidence to support the idea that interferons have an effect on disability progression in PPMS.[34]

What is the best interferon dose?

OVER THE FIRST DECADE OF INTERFERON USE, the general opinion based on trial results and clinical experience was that Betaseron and high-dose Rebif were more or less comparable in terms of their effectiveness, whereas Avonex was the least potent. Despite this, Avonex was more popular in some countries, in large part because a once-weekly injection was easier to take. But why was there any difference among these three very similar drugs? One possibility was that the effectiveness of an interferon was determined either by the dose (i.e. the cumulative amount of drug) or the dosing frequency (i.e. how often it's taken). As a result, many studies looked at dosing issues, which was done primarily for two reasons: to show that one interferon was better than the others; and to explore the possibility that if some drug was good, more drug would be better.

These studies give some idea of how the individual interferons stack up against each other. As we've seen before, the EVIDENCE trial showed that Rebif was superior to Avonex, enabling Rebif to be marketed in the U.S.[22] The other high-profile study was INCOMIN, which compared Betaseron and Avonex.[35] To no one's great surprise, the study found that people taking Betaseron were more likely to have no relapses and had less inflammatory activity on their MRI. A three-way comparison study found that Rebif and Betaseron were about the same, and both were better than Avonex – at least in terms of effectiveness.[36] Despite this, many people still preferred Avonex because of the once-weekly dosing.

Rebif tried to address this preference for less frequent dosing with the OWIMS study, which looked at a once-a-week regimen.[37] The experiment was a bust. Once-weekly Rebif had little effect on relapses, which enabled the investigators to take a parting shot at Avonex, arguing that the results showed that once-weekly interferon regimens were ineffective.[38]

OWIMS was a study of Rebif pretending to be Avonex. A European trial then returned the compliment with a study using twice the usual dose of Avonex ;[39] in effect, this was Avonex pretending to be Rebif. As it turned out, doubling the dose of Avonex wasn't any better than the usual dose, even when the high dose was continued for four years.[40]

Undeterred by the suggestion that more was not better, the OPTIMS study looked at whether a higher dose of Betaseron was worthwhile in people who hadn't responded all that well to the usual dose.[41] The higher dose was better at shutting down inflammation in the brain, but people had a tougher time of it, prompting more in the high-dose group to stop treatment. This was shown again in a trial that used an even higher dose of Betaseron.[42] While it was unclear whether there was a relationship between the dose and the response, there was certainly an association between dose and side effects. Doubling the dose of Betaseron substantially increased the problem of flu-like symptoms, muscle aches and pains, fever, depression, nausea and pain.

All of this jockeying for position accomplished little in terms of how the interferons were perceived or used. The net result of all these internecine squabbles: Rebif and Betaseron were a little more potent, Avonex was easier to take – which is what most people had already known before.

How do the interferons compare to Copaxone?

REBIF ROLLED THE DICE in its comparative trial with Avonex. It rolled them again in a study against Copaxone, no doubt thinking that it would score an easy victory. Copaxone was perceived by many to be of doubtful benefit and was certainly no match for Rebif. That bit of hubris would hurt Rebif and the other interferons immeasurably.

The REGARD study was launched in 2004 and compared people taking Rebif versus Copaxone.[43] After two years, both groups were shown to be doing remarkably well – the number of relapses people had was about one-half of what was expected. But the bigger surprise was that there was no difference between the drugs. People taking Copaxone didn't relapse any sooner than those on Rebif. The MRI picture was very similar with the two drugs, which went against the general thinking that Rebif would at least be better at reducing inflammation in the brain. A possible explanation was that the people in the trial didn't have active enough disease for Rebif to demonstrate its greater potency, but this interpretation didn't gain much support.

Next up was Betaseron, which followed up its BENEFIT study with a brace of "BE" studies called BECOME and BEYOND. BECOME compared standard doses of Betaseron and Copaxone and found they had comparable effects on MRI measures of disease activity.[44] BEYOND doubled-down by comparing both the standard dose and twice the usual dose of Betaseron with standard-dose Copaxone;[45] "BEYOND" presumably referred to dosing rather than credulity. There was no advantage with high-dose Betaseron compared to Copaxone with respect to any of the measures studied – relapse risk, disability progression or MRI measures. However, there were disadvantages. About 50% more people stopped taking high-dose Betaseron compared to standard-dose Betaseron, presumably because they were having problems tolerating the side effects associated with this higher dose.

So the mad gamble of comparing interferons with Copaxone didn't pay off. The net result was that people changed their opinion about the relative merits of the injectable MS drugs. Interferons were much the same; and Copaxone was no worse. This may have helped the popularity of Copaxone, which in some countries became the most-prescribed drug for people newly diagnosed with MS.

Are interferons equally effective in everyone?

MS AFFECTS PEOPLE DIFFERENTLY, so perhaps it isn't surprising that MS drugs may affect people in somewhat different ways. MS is more common in women; when men get MS, they are at greater risk of having a more severe, progressive course.[46] Although most people studied in clinical trials of MS drugs are women, it's generally assumed that there's no difference in how treatment affects women and men. This may or may not be true. One study found that men treated with an interferon were less likely to have a relapse on treatment compared to women, however, they were also more likely to have progression of disability.[47] In contrast, an analysis of people enrolled in Avonex clinical trials found no difference in how men and women respond to an interferon.[48]

If there are differences in drug response, it may be because the immune system works somewhat differently in men and women.[49,50] It may also be that men are more likely to develop antibodies to interferon, which neutralize the effect of the drug,[51] but this needs to be studied further.

MS primarily affects women of northern European descent, which influences who is enrolled in drug trials, and so there is little information on the effects of interferons (or other drugs) in different ethnic groups. For example, of the 301 people in the initial Avonex trial, only 20 were black (i.e. about 7%).[17] The situation is no better today. In the DEFINE trial of Tecfidera (dimethyl fumarate), only 26 people (2%) were black.[52]

So although MS is known to have a more severe course in African-Americans,[53] there is limited evidence about the effectiveness of interferons (or any other drug) in this group. Only two studies have looked at this question. An analysis of people in the EVIDENCE trial comparing Rebif and Avonex found that African-Americans had more relapses and more disease activity on their MRI compared to whites, suggesting that interferons are somewhat less effective.[54] It's important to note, however, that this conclusion was based on a very small number of African-Americans (36 in total) compared to the number of whites in the study (616).

The only other study compared how well African-Americans and whites did during treatment with an interferon.[55] Overall, blacks had more rapid disability progression than whites, suggesting that they didn't respond equally well to treatment or that the interferon was unequal to the task of controlling their more severe symptoms.

There are few studies of interferons in other ethnic groups. One small study in Bangalore reported that interferons are effective in Indians;[56] and a study in Hong Kong suggested that treatment may be less effective in Asians.[57] But since large clinical trials are typically conducted in Europe or North America – in large part because of the higher prevalence of MS in these two regions – there is limited information on the use of MS drugs in other ethnic groups.

What are the side effects of the interferons?

SINCE INTERFERON IS PRODUCED by cells to combat viruses, perhaps it isn't surprising that one of the more difficult side effects of interferon treatment is flu-like symptoms. Up to 75% of people taking an interferon will experience flu-like symptoms[58] – making them more of an effect inherent to the drug rather than a side effect (cold comfort to anyone taking them). Flu-like symptoms can include muscle aches, chills, sweating and headache accompanied by fever. Taking a painkiller, such as ibuprofen (Motrin, Advil) or acetaminophen (Tylenol or Panadol; also known as paracetemol), before the injection can make these symptoms a bit more tolerable.[59,60] It's often said that flu-like symptoms diminish if you stay on therapy and this may be true in some cases. But many people find that the problem drags on and never really goes away,[61] which can make it a real challenge to tough it out on treatment.

An even more common problem is skin reactions at the site where you inject yourself. According to the most recent estimate, skin reactions occur in about 90% – or pretty much everyone who takes an interferon.[62] Since the reaction is due to the injection itself, there's no way to avoid this side effect. Some studies have suggested that injection-site reactions are less common with Avonex compared to the other interferons; this is because the drug is injected deep into the muscle rather than just under the skin. The trade-off is that injecting into the muscle can be a more intimidating prospect for some, and may be more painful. Pain and skin reactions at the injection site are generally mild, but they can be severe and persistent in some people. Injection-site reactions are one of the most common reasons why people stop taking their interferon or switch to another drug.[63]

Over the short and longer term, interferons are considered to be very safe,[64] but some nasty side effects can occur. Interferons can cause liver problems, so regular blood tests are needed to monitor liver function. The most serious cases of liver damage have occurred in people with pre-existing liver disease. Combining interferons with alcohol is also very hard on the liver and should be avoided.

In some people, liver damage will be due to autoimmune hepatitis. Indeed, it's often overlooked that interferon use may be associated with a variety of autoimmune flare-ups that can cause problems. The thyroid, a gland in the neck that plays an important role in body metabolism, appears to be especially vulnerable to the effect of interferons (as well as to Lemtrada, as we'll see). A one-year study reported that thyroid dysfunction occurred in one in three people with MS treated with an interferon.[65] While most people didn't develop any symptoms, thyroid function should be regularly monitored with blood tests during interferon therapy, especially in those with a family history of thyroid disease.[66]

These concerns aside, the greatest challenge for people on an interferon is weathering the flu-ish symptoms and skin reactions. Interferons have been a mainstay of MS treatment for almost two decades, but they are not well loved. Numerous studies have found that people try to stick with the program for a while, but many – about 40-50% – give up after two or three years.[67-70] The reasons for this are many: flu-like symptoms drag them down, they don't like the frequent injections, or they don't believe that medication is helping their MS. In the MS Choices study, many people simply said they were "emotionally/mentally drained" and "fed up with the treatment".[71]

We'll return to this issue in the last chapter when we talk about some of the things to consider when choosing the best treatment for your MS.

CHAPTER 6

WHAT IS COPAXONE?

IN THE 1960S, a great deal of work on the immune system was being performed at the Weizmann Institute in Israel, a research centre founded in 1934 by chemist Chaim Weizmann, who would later become the first president of Israel. A particular interest was long chains of amino acids, the building blocks of proteins. The researchers found they could induce an immune response to these substances, and this immunogenicity extended to other molecules bound up in the polymer, including lipids (fats).[1] It occurred to the scientists that a matrix of proteins and lipids was very similar in structure to myelin, the fatty sheath that insulates nerve fibres. Myelin proteins are the antigens that are attacked by the body's own immune system in MS, so it seemed that the protein-lipid polymer (or copolymer) might be useful for studying MS.

MS doesn't develop in animals. So to understand the process of demyelination, researchers use an animal model called experimental autoimmune encephalomyelitis. EAE is a condition created in the laboratory in which animals are injected with brain or spinal cord tissue, which causes a rapidly progressing form of demyelination. This phenomenon was first described in the 1930s by scientists investigating the demyelination that can occur with rabies vaccine,[2] but it was only three decades later that researchers identified that one of the myelin proteins (called myelin basic protein, or MBP) could induce EAE.[3] When MBP was injected, the body detected it as a foreign protein and attacked it, then subsequently attacked the body's own MBP, which stripped the myelin from the nerve fibres. In other words, MBP could be used as an antigen to induce an antibody response.

The Weizmann researchers reasoned that their own synthetic amino acid-lipid copolymer might be useful as a way of inducing EAE in guinea pigs (the literal kind). Over the course of a year, various formulations were injected to induce an immune reaction. All of the experiments failed.[4] They thought about giving up on the project, but decided to try one last experiment. As it turned out, instead of causing EAE, the copolymer actually suppressed its development. Among the compounds tested, the most active was the first, Copolymer-1, which was made up of a random assortment of amino acids: Glutamic acid, Lysine, Alanine and Tyrosine. Their initials, GLAT, would become glatiramer acetate. It would later be branded as Copaxone – which combined the Cop of copolymer with axone (or nerve fibre).

Copaxone suppressed the development of EAE not only in guinea pigs, but also in rabbits, mice, monkeys and baboons,[1] so the thought was that it might work in humans as well. Another observation was that Copaxone's effects appeared to be specific to demyelinating diseases. There was no effect in other autoimmune disorders.

The next step was to test the drug in humans. A pilot study in Israel found that Copaxone had little effect in four people with advanced MS. A larger pilot study in Germany subsequently found that there was some improvement in people with earlier-stage MS. Then a preliminary study and two pilot studies in the U.S. were encouraging enough to launch a larger phase II placebo-controlled trial.[5-7] Over the course of two years, people who injected Copaxone experienced fewer relapses than those in the placebo group, and twice as many taking Copaxone had no relapses at all.

These results were unprecedented at the time, but when the researchers tried to peddle Cop-1 to drug companies such as Johnson & Johnson and Upjohn, no one was interested. To a company like Johnson & Johnson, which sold Tylenol, or Upjohn, which manufactured Motrin (and later Rogaine), MS was too small a market and Cop-1 was a niche product. But a company in Israel, Teva (Hebrew for Nature), saw the potential and a deal was struck in 1987 – fully 20 years after the Weizmann researchers first began to study Copaxone.

How does Copaxone work?

COPAXONE – LIKE THE INTERFERONS BEFORE IT – was a wrongheaded idea that ended up being a treatment for MS. It didn't cause EAE, the demyelinating disease in experimental animals, but actually suppressed it. How it suppressed EAE and why it seemed to work in MS are still the subjects of debate.

As discussed in Chapter 1, autoreactive T cells attack myelin proteins such as MBP. Copaxone resembles MBP, and the researchers initially believed that Copaxone was similar enough that T cells attacked the drug instead of MBP.[1] This bait-and-switch is called molecular mimicry (previously discussed in the context of viruses). Molecular mimicry may be why the body mistakenly thinks myelin proteins are viral proteins.[8,9] This has been shown for a number of viral strains such as coronavirus (which can cause colds and respiratory diseases, including SARS [sudden acute respiratory syndrome]), which is cross-reactive with MBP.[10] This means that a coronavirus infection has the potential to activate the inflammatory immune response directed at myelin in people with MS. This mimicry is not limited to one virus – various viruses (notably Epstein-Barr) and bacteria have been suggested as possible triggers of MS.[11,12] And once the immune response is activated by a specific antigen, it can react to similar antigens through epitope spreading.

So if the immune system is fooled into thinking that its target is a viral protein (but is actually the body's own myelin), Copaxone may fool immune cells into thinking it's the target. However, when the T cells encounter Copaxone molecules, there isn't the usual release of inflammatory substances that damages tissues in the CNS. The immune system is ready to start a fire; Copaxone resembles a match but doesn't produce a flame.

Molecular mimicry was an attractive hypothesis, but later research suggested that it might not be the whole answer. Studies in animals showed that Copaxone could suppress EAE induced by myelin proteins other than MBP,[13-15] so the theory was revised. T-helper cells of the immune system will respond differently depending on the antigen they encounter. As mentioned before, the Th1 subtype promotes inflammation whereas the Th2 subtype suppresses inflammation. The new idea was that Copaxone still acted as an antigen and was taken up by immune cells (antigen-presenting cells, or APCs). But when APCs presented Copaxone to T cells, the Th cells developed into the Th2 type and released cytokines to suppress inflammation (rather than the Th1 type, which promotes inflammation). In the brain, this tolerance to MBP could extend to other myelin proteins so there was a less robust immune response to myelin. This is called bystander suppression.[16-18] Such a mechanism is necessary when you're trying to suppress an immune reaction and you don't know what the target is (i.e. what is the antigen triggering the immune response). So it was suggested that Copaxone covered all bases, inducing a less damaging immune response to all of the myelin proteins.

How effective is Copaxone in treating RRMS?

THE INITIAL PHASE II STUDY PUBLISHED in 1987 appeared very promising, but it didn't provide enough evidence that Copaxone was safe and effective. Larger studies were needed. The first challenge for researchers was to produce enough of the drug. Each batch was only enough to treat a thousand people for one day, and large-scale production was needed – a process that took another two years.[1]

An open-label study was completed in Israel, then a large placebo-controlled study involving 251 people with MS was launched at 11 centres in the U.S.[19] Over the course of the two-year study, people taking Copaxone had an average of 1.29 relapses per person (adjusted mean 1.19) compared to 1.67 per person in the placebo group (adjusted mean 1.68). This represented a 29% (unadjusted 23%) reduction in the relapse rate with Copaxone. What this means is that treatment reduced relapse frequency by a little less than one-third.

The researchers claimed there was effect on disability progression, but there wasn't, at least not according to how these things are usually measured. From one visit to the next over a three-month period, a similar proportion of people on treatment or placebo showed a sustained change in EDSS. Over three-quarters of the people in both groups showed no progression.

The phase II study and this phase III trial (called pivotal or registration studies because they were intended for submission to regulatory authorities) provided the basis for Copaxone's approval by the FDA as an MS treatment in December 1996. The drug was approved to reduce the frequency of MS relapses; a claim for reducing disability progression was rejected by the FDA. Re-calculations of the phase III data suggested there was some benefit on progression,[20] but the FDA remained unconvinced.

One major shortcoming of the phase III trial was that no MRIs were done because imaging wasn't considered to be standard practice at the time the study was being designed. This was a considerable disadvantage in the increasingly competitive MS market. The pivotal interferon-beta trials had shown that they had an effect on MRI lesions, which gave the impression that they were more effective. A small MRI study of Copaxone was done as a stop-gap,[21] followed a year later by a larger international study. In the European/Canadian

MRI trial, 239 people with MS were randomized to Copaxone or placebo and received monthly MRIs for nine months.[22] Although the study period was very short, Copaxone did show that it reduced the number and size of inflammatory lesions in the brain.

The key Copaxone trials didn't end after the predetermined study period – a common phenomenon of MS studies. They continued as extension studies in which everyone – including those initially on placebo – received the active therapy. In part this was to offset the complaint that two- or three-year studies aren't really representative of what happens during the life-long course of MS.

For the extension of the pivotal trial, MRI measures were added to make up for the original oversight. While this was intended as a way of bolstering the MRI argument, extension studies can't really demonstrate efficacy because everyone is on treatment – so there's nothing to compare to the treatment. The only comparator is time: people in the placebo group started treatment two years later than those initially randomized to the Copaxone group. So the extension data can hint at whether people are worse off if treatment is delayed. People on treatment for the longer period – about six years – were somewhat better off than those on treatment for only four years with respect to relapses and MRI findings.[23] However, the researchers concluded that the effects of Copaxone on MRI lesions were modest at best.[23]

One of the key problems of extension studies is that some people originally enrolled in the study may decide not to participate, and this was the case in the Copaxone study. Of the 239 in the initial study, only 147 – or 62% – continued on long-term treatment. And

MRI scans were only done on 135 people, or just over one-half of the original sample. This drop in numbers gives a diminishing return with respect to how the results can be interpreted. What happened to everyone who dropped out of the study? Were the drop-outs in the Copaxone group or the placebo group? Were they so happy with treatment that they decided to leave the study, or so unhappy? As for those who continued on treatment, it may be reasonable to think that they were a self-selected group – they were doing well so they wanted to stay on therapy.

In fact this appears to have been the case. If you look at the people in the Copaxone trial who dropped out, most had started to progress and they were having more relapses compared to those who kept taking the drug.[24] The drug wasn't working for them – so they quit taking it.

Over the past decade, there has been a steady drip-drip of data from the long-term extensions of both the Copaxone pivotal trial and the European/Canadian MRI trial. The pivotal study published updates at three, six, eight, 10, 15 and 20 years after the start of the trial.[25-30] After 20 years there were only 74 people still in the study – the other 78% of the subjects had wandered off to parts unknown. Those who had stayed with therapy were doing well as you might expect – relapse rates were low and two-thirds hadn't progressed to secondary-progressive MS (EDSS 4) after 27 years of living with MS. So that was a remarkable achievement.

Can this good news be attributed to Copaxone? That's a little more uncertain. The frequency of relapses normally decreases during the course of MS even without treatment. The people still on therapy may have represented a group of people who had responded especially well to Copaxone (sometimes called "super-responders"), or they may have been people without aggressive MS. It's hard to tell. What can be said about these long-term studies is that Copaxone appears to be very safe. The side effects during long-term use were the same as those seen during short-term use – there were no surprises. There was no evidence suggesting that Copaxone damaged the liver or kidneys, or caused the development of other autoimmune diseases or cancers.

Can Copaxone be used in people without RRMS?

SINCE COPAXONE WAS APPROVED for use in RRMS, two key studies have looked at whether it's effective in people with different levels of disease severity.

As discussed in Chapter 2, CIS is diagnosed when a person has early signs of neurological problems but doesn't meet the full criteria for a diagnosis of MS.[31] The first study to look at whether treatment was beneficial in CIS appeared in 2000,[32] and CIS became a hot area of research. At the time, it was bruited that earlier treatment might be better able to prevent some of the damage that occurs in MS, much as you want to treat an infection early before it gets out of control. CIS was an early sign that something was amiss, so the hope was that treating CIS might delay the development of full-blown MS (or at least a full-blown diagnosis of MS).

The Avonex trial in CIS showed that treatment could delay a second MS-like attack, and so CIS trials were launched for most of the MS drugs. The last in the series was the Copaxone trial, called PreCISe, which combined CIS and a hint of it being pre-MS in one title.[33] This large study, which enrolled 481 people in 16 countries, found that Copaxone was significantly better than a placebo, delaying the development of MS by about a year in one-quarter of the subjects. As a result, the FDA approved the use of Copaxone in people with CIS in February 2009.

Less successful was PROMise, the trial of Copaxone in people with primary-progressive MS.[34] While Copaxone seemed to provide some benefit in men, overall it wasn't effective in treating PPMS. In this it was no different than any of the other MS drugs: none has been shown to be effective in PPMS. This continues to be the greatest disappointment of all to people living with progressive MS, and the great failure of MS research thus far. Copaxone hasn't been studied in secondary-progressive MS. So Copaxone is not approved for use either in people with primary- or secondary-progressive MS.

Why does Copaxone have to be injected?

COPAXONE IS A RANDOM assortment of amino acids, which are the building blocks of proteins. Proteins are fragile molecules and very susceptible to breakdown by stomach acids, so often they can't be administered orally.. In contrast, pharmaceutical chemicals are often not destroyed by stomach acid, or can be produced with a protective covering (such as a capsule) or formulated so that the active ingredients are released only after they have passed through the stomach.

An attempt was made to develop an oral formulation of Copaxone. The idea behind it was that much of the body's immune tissue can be found in the gastrointestinal tract, and exposure to antigens (such as Copaxone) can induce what is called oral tolerance: after an initial exposure, the immune system responds less robustly to subsequent exposures.[35] In fact, one of the first MS treatments – oral myelin – tested this idea two decades ago at Harvard University in people with MS (the treatment failed[36]).

Oral Copaxone did appear to have an effect on the immune system when it was tested in animals.[37] Unfortunately, a very large trial of oral Copaxone, called CORAL, was a failure. The oral formulation of Copaxone had no effect on relapse or other measures of MS activity.[38] Only the injectable form has any claim to effectiveness.

Is one injection a day the best dosing?

ALL OF THE EARLY STUDIES of Copaxone used the dose of 20 mg injected once a day,[1] which was was a little unusual. Dose-finding studies are often done in the early days of clinical research to determine the lowest effective dose of a drug so as to minimize drug exposure, toxicities and side effects. This wasn't done for Copaxone. All of the clinical trials studied only the 20 mg dose.

Making use of the rationale that a little is good and more is better (a concept that doesn't necessarily apply to immune-active drugs), a higher dose of Copaxone was studied. Preliminary results from the 9006 trial showed that 40 mg of Copaxone was no more effective than 20 mg.[39] Apparently not satisfied with this answer, the question was posed again in a phase III trial.[40] In the FORTE study, over 1,100 people received either the standard dose of Copaxone (20 mg once-daily) or twice that dose for one year. There was no benefit when the dose of Copaxone was doubled. But side effects were more common with the higher dose, as you would expect.

Of course this doesn't establish if 20 mg once-daily is the best dose. In fact, two studies have looked at whether reducing the dose makes any difference. An open-label study found that injecting every other day instead of every day didn't appear to make much difference.[41] Another found that taking the usual 20-mg dose of Copaxone – but injecting it only twice a week – did not alter the effectiveness with respect to reducing the rate of relapses or the risk of disability.[42] Fewer injections, not surprisingly, were associated with fewer injection-related problems.

These two strategies – higher dose, less frequent injections – were combined in the GALA (Glatiramer Acetate Low frequency Administration) study of Copaxone 40 mg administered three times a week.[43] Treatment reduced relapses by one-third, similar to what's seen with the usual regimen. While these results indicated that different dosing schemes may work, some have speculated that the real goal of GALA was to allow a new application to the FDA that would extend the patent life of Copaxone.[44] If so, the strategy was effective for this regimen of three times per week was indeed approved by the FDA in 2014.

Although Copaxone dosing appears to be flexible, this isn't to suggest that you should reduce the dosing that your doctor has prescribed. What it does mean, however, is that it probably isn't the end of the world if you forget to take one of your daily injections – it won't have an effect on your MS. And if you're having problems taking the drug because of injection site reactions or other problems, talk to your doctor about reducing the frequency of your injections, at least for a time.

The question of Copaxone dosing raises an interesting (admittedly theoretical) question: Is Copaxone a drug, or is it a vaccine? In other words, is regular, perhaps daily treatment with Copaxone needed to control the MS disease process? Or does it work like a vaccine, so after the initial series of injections, all you need are periodic booster shots? The idea that Copaxone is actually a vaccine was proposed a decade ago,[45] and included the thought that different dosing might be appropriate if a person enters the progressive phase of MS when neurodegeneration predominates. Unfortunately, studies to investigate this possibility have not been done and it's unlikely they'll be undertaken.

What side effects can I expect with Copaxone?

COPAXONE IS A VERY SAFE medication and is not generally associated with serious side effects. The most common side effect is skin reactions at the site where you inject yourself; reactions can include redness, swelling, rash and pain. Injection reactions were the most common reason why people stopped taking Copaxone in clinical trials.

The most alarming symptom with Copaxone is called an immediate post-injection reaction. This can feel like a feeling of panic, difficulty catching your breath, flushing and chest pain – as if you're having a heart attack. It's extremely uncomfortable (and worrisome), however, the effect soon subsides and isn't associated with any long-term problems. It's not a heart attack, it doesn't mean you're having a panic attack, and it doesn't mean you're going crazy. This reaction just comes at you out of nowhere, and gets better on its own. It was once felt that this side effect was more common after being on treatment for a few months, but it's now known that it can happen at any time – even after years of treatment. The cause of it is unknown.

A bigger problem is lipoatrophy – denting and pitting of the skin that resembles cellulite. This can be quite disfiguring and many people find it very upsetting when they first notice it. Skin pitting was reported in the initial trial of Copaxone but was said at the time to persist for only a few days. The true extent of the problem was only realized in 1999 after a letter appeared in a dermatology journal.[46] While initially considered to be a mere clinical curiosity, a scant two years later it was recognized that many – if not most – people taking Copaxone were developing this problem.[47] Pitting of the skin is caused by a loss of fat tissue below the surface of the skin, and this can occur with subcutaneous injections of many different medications (or even with acupuncture). What makes lipoatrophy a potentially bigger problem during Copaxone use is the frequency of injections. It occurs almost exclusively in women, and is especially common in those with fair or red hair.[47] Several studies have shown that it's more likely to occur with injections in the thighs and arms and less likely when you inject into the abdomen.[46-48]

The best treatment for lipoatrophy is prevention. If pitting develops on one part of the body, avoid injecting that site again for a while. Re-injection may make it worse. Rotate the sites of injection – upper arm, thigh, abdomen, etc. – to lower the risk of lipoatrophy.

There are no established treatments for lipoatrophy. The problem may diminish or improve when Copaxone is stopped,[49] although one case has been reported of progressive lipoatrophy even after the drug was stopped.[50] Lipoatrophy appears to come back again if Copaxone is re-started, so another treatment may be better if you find this side effect to be troublesome.

CHAPTER **7**

WHAT IS TYSABRI?

THE FIRST MS THERAPIES were the products of serendipity rather than of design. But as more was learned about the abnormal immune response in MS throughout the 1990s, researchers started thinking about ways to interfere with this process. Attention focused on the activated T cells that invaded the brain and spinal cord, resulting in the inflammation and nerve damage that are the hallmarks of MS.

For T cells to enter the central nervous system, they first have to adhere to the tightly packed cells that form the blood-brain barrier. After attaching themselves to this barrier, the T cells then squeeze through and enter the brain and spinal cord. One way to slow down or stop this process is to disable the adhesion molecules that allow the T cells to stick to the blood-brain barrier.

A key player in this process is an adhesion molecule called alpha-4 integrin,[1] which is found mostly on immune cells, such as T and B cells. Alpha-4 integrin resembles a lollipop with the sticky end projecting out from the surface of the immune cell. This enables the T cell to stick to the inner lining of blood vessels – the first step in the invasion of the CNS.

To prevent this, researchers developed a monoclonal antibody (or MAb) that targets the alpha-4 integrin protein. A MAb is a biological therapy (rather than a pharmaceutical or drug). To produce a MAb, researchers create antibody-producing cells from a single original cell. These cells are clones (i.e. genetically identical) and are called monoclonal because of their sole common ancestor. Originally these MAbs were produced by combining myeloma cells (a type of cancer affecting white blood cells, used because they keep dividing indefinitely) with spleen cells (which produce antibodies) from a mouse or rabbit. So in effect, you turn the cancer cell into a factory that can produce antibodies on an industrial scale. However, this can create problems because a mouse antibody is not the same as a human antibody and the immune system can tell the difference. So human and mouse are often combined using recombinant techniques to produce a "humanized" MAb that is partly human and partly mouse.

This technology has led to the development of dozens of monoclonal antibodies used in medicine today – identifiable by the *mab* suffix. Examples are infliximab for rheumatoid arthritis, and the anti-cancer drugs bevacizumab and trastuzumab. As we'll see later on, the first MAb that later became an MS drug was alemtuzumab (Lemtrada, see Chapter 12). Other MAbs in development for MS are daclizumab, ocrelizumab and ofatumumab. Each of these MAbs has been developed for a very specific target.

The first MAb to make it to market as an MS treatment was natalizumab (Tysabri). Originally produced in mouse myeloma cells in the 1980s, it is a recombinant humanized MAb that targets the alpha-4 integrin protein. In effect, it acts as a wrapper to cover the sticky lollipop so activated T cells can't adhere to the blood-brain barrier and invade the CNS. So natalizumab is the first "designer" therapy in MS. Like most biological therapies, natalizumab has to be administered by intravenous infusion (a slow drip into the body).

Preliminary studies in an animal model of MS found that this novel approach to treatment could indeed slow the accumulation of activated T cells in the CNS.[2] A phase I safety study and a phase II trial in humans were both published in 1999.[3,4]

The results from the phase II study were very promising. After two infusions given a month apart, people receiving natalizumab showed a 50% reduction in new MS brain lesions. One other finding in this study would also become important later on: once the infusions were stopped, people in the natalizumab group quickly lost any benefit. Brain lesions reappeared and relapses became more frequent compared to what was seen in the placebo group. It wasn't clear if this recurrence of disease activity was a return to how things had been before, or a "rebound effect" in which the disease becomes worse than before. This would become (and still is) a hot topic of debate.

A larger study (Study 231) of natalizumab soon followed.[5] People received one of two doses of natalizumab (3 or 6 milligrams per kilogram of body weight, e.g. a person weighing 50 kg [110 pounds] would receive either 150 or 300 mg of the drug) or a placebo every 28 days for six months. The main goal was to look at the ongoing effect of the drug on MRI lesions, although the impact on relapses was also assessed. The number of new lesions was substantially lower with natalizumab – about one new lesion per person compared to almost 10 per person in the placebo group. There were also fewer relapses with treatment compared to placebo.

The results of this phase II study generated a great deal of excitement. Thus far, the development of natalizumab had proceeded at an extraordinary pace and the speed of events would soon accelerate. Natalizumab was fast-tracked by the FDA and in November 2004 – fewer than two years after the phase II study and before any phase III studies were published – it received approval as an MS treatment. Its brand name, Antegren, was rejected by the FDA because it was too similar to other brands such as Ativan (used to treat anxiety) and Integrilin (for heart disease). So the new name became Tysabri.

The reason for this rapid approval – less than six months from submission to approval – was the feeling that Tysabri was appreciably better than the injectable therapies already on the market. Doctors quickly adopted the new drug and sales were expected to top $2 billion a year. However, as with all blockbuster drugs, more sales means that more people are being exposed to the drug and that is when previously unknown side effects crop up.

In the headlong drive to make Tysabri the top MS drug, the wheels were quick to fall off. A scant three months later, in February 2005, Tysabri was withdrawn from the market.

What happened?

The ostensible problem was an infection called progressive multifocal leukoencephalopathy (PML; see below for an explanation). But other issues were also in play. The first and most obvious was that Tysabri was approved too quickly by the FDA. In fact, the two key trials of the drug had not yet been published. Some details had been presented at international meetings, but the full results had not appeared in print and had not been discussed and debated by the medical community.

Approval was based on preliminary results only.[6] Study 1801, which would later be known as the AFFIRM trial (for Antegren Safety and Efficacy in Relapsing Remitting MS), was a two-year study but only one year's worth of data were available to the FDA. Study 1802, later called SENTINEL (for Safety and Efficacy of Natalizumab in combination with Interferon Beta-1a in Patients with Relapsing Remitting MS), was also planned as a two-year study but only one year of data were available (and only year of data would ultimately appear). Both of these phase III trials were published in 2006 – over a year after Tysabri had already been withdrawn.

In its initial approval of Tysabri, the FDA admitted that it wasn't sure that one year of benefit was clinically meaningful;[6] all of the other MS drugs had shown a two-year benefit. But the bureaucrats decided that a one-year benefit would serve as a surrogate for a two-year benefit. Since a reduction in relapses is in itself a surrogate endpoint (meaning it's a stand-in for a benefit rather than a direct effect on the disease), the FDA had put itself in a position of approving a drug based on a surrogate of a surrogate – an unprecedented move from a government agency, even one with the FDA's somewhat chequered past.

Another oddity was dosing. Tysabri was initially tested in humans using doses based on body weight (3 or 6 milligrams per kilogram, with the higher dose providing no additional benefit). By the time the two phase III trials rolled around, that dose had become a one-size-fits-all 300 mg. This presumed that the average MS patient – a women in her 20s or 30s – taking the lower dose weighed 100 kg (220 pounds). This meant that people were being unnecessarily exposed to more drug than they needed and more side effects than they wanted. Indeed, the FDA noted that the 300 mg dose might be given less frequently and still be effective,[6] a strategy that would re-emerge almost a decade later.

The quickie approval also had more obvious safety implications. The FDA review was based on data for 1,617 people who had been exposed to Tysabri for a median of 20 months, a rather short time given that it was intended for people with a life-long disease. But the FDA deemed this sufficient, and ruled that no specific risk management activities were required. Accordingly, the product monograph warned doctors only about the risk of hypersensitivity reactions (such as rash, flushing and difficulty breathing) that can occur in the first few hours after a Tysabri infusion.[7] No other safety issues were flagged by the FDA in its review of the preliminary data. The deaths that had occurred during trials (a total of six in people exposed to the drug) didn't appear to be related to Tysabri.

But that was before PML emerged.

What is PML?

PROGRESSIVE MULTIFOCAL LEUKOENCEPHALOPATHY (PML) is a rare disease that was first reported in 1958.[8] As the name implies, it's a widespread (i.e. more than one focus) brain disorder that causes inflammation and tissue damage in the white matter of the brain ("leuko" meaning white, "encephalo" meaning brain, "patho" meaning disease). Symptoms can include headaches, seizures, impaired thinking and speech, loss of eyesight, and difficulty walking.[9] In many cases it's fatal; for most people it produces terrible disability.

In 1971, a new virus was isolated in a PML patient named John Cunningham,[10] and he received the dubious honour of having the JC virus named after him. Initially, PML was seen mostly in people with blood cancers, but even so it was exceedingly rare: by 1984, only 69 cases had been confirmed worldwide.[9] A few cases of PML were then seen in people with the condition that would later become known as AIDS.[11] Over the next 15 years, people with AIDS would account for 87% of all PML deaths.[12]

The JC virus (JCV) is everywhere. Most people encounter it by late adolescence, and about 90% show exposure at some point in their lifetime.[13] It isn't known how JCV is transmitted but some have suggested that the source may be food or drinking water.[14] Initially, the virus is believed to infect the tonsils,[15] although it generally doesn't cause any symptoms. The virus then moves in to stay, living primarily in the kidneys, lymph nodes and bone marrow.[16,17] JCV can infect various tissues. However, it can only reproduce if it invades the tonsils, certain immune cells (including B cells, which produce antibodies), and cells in the brain, such as oligodendrocytes (which produce myelin). So these are the key reservoirs of viral activity.

Most people aren't aware that they have been exposed to JCV; their immune systems appear to keep the virus in check. However, a problem can develop if the body's immune surveillance is impaired.

This allows the virus to be reactivated – which occurs almost exclusively when a person becomes immunocompromised either because of a disease (such as AIDS or lymphoma) or from taking an immunosuppressing drug (such as chemotherapy or an anti-rejection drug). A similar viral reactivation phenomenon is seen with shingles, in which the long-dormant herpes zoster virus becomes active.

How JCV gets into the brain isn't entirely clear. The most likely way is the Trojan horse strategy: the virus infects a cell (such as a B cell or stem cell) in the body, then hitches a ride when the cell enters the brain.[18] Another suggestion is that the virus can lie dormant in oligodendrocytes in the brain until conditions are right. The presence of JCV in the brain doesn't appear to be an actual trigger for MS. When researchers examined MS lesions, none contained active JCV,[19] so it isn't considered one of the possible viruses that may initiate the MS disease process.

As JCV divides in the brain, the body reacts by producing extensive inflammation that can be seen with an MRI. While the pattern of inflammation is different from what is seen in MS, the two can be confused, especially if someone isn't looking for PML.

Tysabri and PML

FOLLOWING THE REPORT OF TWO DEATHS of people treated with Tysabri, the drug was withdrawn from the market by the manufacturer, Biogen Idec. One death occurred in someone with MS in the SENTINEL trial, which combined Tysabri and Avonex. The thinking was that this double hit of immunosuppression promoted

JCV reactivation. The case involved a 46-year-old woman from Colorado, who was diagnosed with PML after receiving 37 monthly doses of Tysabri.[20] In December 2004 she developed neurological and cognitive problems; her doctors assumed she was experiencing a worsening of her MS, so she was given two courses of steroids. Her condition deteriorated rapidly, and she died in February 2005. A second case in SENTINEL involved a 44-year-old man in California who developed severe cognitive problems after receiving 28 monthly infusions of Tysabri. His symptoms progressed rapidly and at the lowest point he was confined to his bed and was unable to communicate. While he did survive and later showed some improvement, at last report he was still partially paralysed, had disabling ataxia (inability to coordinate muscle movements) and cognitive impairment.[21]

The second death was a 60-year-old man in Belgium enrolled in a trial of Tysabri for Crohn's disease (the drug's other development track). His death in 2003 was initially attributed to a brain tumour but was later determined to be due to PML. He received just eight infusions of Tysabri.[22]

A sad irony to this story is that the first person with MS to die from PML probably didn't have MS at all,[23-25] raising unsettling questions about how carefully people are selected for drug trials.[23]

Manufacturers Biogen Idec were quick to respond – to their credit. They withdrew the drug and suspended all trials in MS and Crohn's disease. New data were presented at the annual meeting of the American Academy of Neurology two months later in Miami, but the planned celebration proved to be more of a wake. As one researcher put it: "There was a general air of disappointment that natalizumab had, necessarily, needed to be withdrawn".[26] In its short life, Tysabri had won over a lot of supporters and they were reluctant to give up on the drug.

PML taught an important lesson: there were important, sometimes fatal, risks associated with treating MS. Were those risks worth it? This was the beginning of the central issue in MS therapeutics today: Are the benefits of treatment enough to justify the risks?

The answer is clearly no if the benefits are uncertain and the risks seem high (the FDA's initial take on Lemtrada). For Tysabri the benefits were there. So the next step was to better quantify the risks to make the benefit-risk calculation more defined, and reassure doctors enough to prescribe it. Which is what Tysabri's manufacturers did.

Researchers combed through the database of some three thousand people exposed to Tysabri for about 18 months and found no additional cases of PML.[27] Their rough estimate was that the risk of developing PML was one in a thousand. In subsequent years, as the number of people on Tysabri increased, there was a corresponding increase in the number of people with PML. But the original back-of-the-envelope estimate remained at one in a thousand. Unfortunately, as tens of thousands of people have been exposed to the drug, this low incidence of PML translates to an alarming number of people who have developed a devastating disease. The number of PML cases leapfrogged from 159 (September 2011[28]) to 271 cases (August 2012[29]), then to 472 cases (July 2014[30]), including over 100 deaths. At last report (December 2014), there were 517 cases.[31] What was once rare no longer is. There is little doubt that these figures underestimate the true number of people with PML.

People who survive PML have a variety of severe problems and generally require full-time care. The rate of new cases (about 10 per month) is now over two-fold higher than it was two years ago. This is believed to be because of the growing use of Tysabri rather than a change in risk, although other factors may be involved.

Thus far, three key factors are known to increase the risk of developing PML: taking Tysabri for more than two years; having received prior treatment with an immunosuppressant drug (e.g. mitoxantrone [Novantrone], azathioprine [Imuran], methotrexate, cyclophosphamide or mycophenolate [Cellcept]); and having been exposed to JCV (i.e. if you're antibody-positive). But it's important to emphasize that these are the factors that are known – they are not the only risk factors (since there is some risk of PML, however low, even if all three are absent). These other risk factors aren't well established.

If you have none of these known risk factors, the chance of developing PML is reportedly about 1 in 1,000.[32] This may seem low, but it is 10-fold higher than the original estimate. If you have all of the risk factors, the estimated risk of developing PML is 10 times higher, or about 1% (1.3 per 100)[32] – which may be too high a risk for many people with these risk factors given how devastating PML can be. So it's becoming increasing common for doctors to stop Tysabri once people have totted up one or two risk factors, such as JCV antibody-positivity and/or twenty-four monthly doses of the drug.

The return of Tysabri

PUTTING NUMBERS TO THE PML RISK, however approximate they were, was reassuring to many people and emboldened them to readopt Tysabri when it became available again. The potential benefits became clearer when the two pivotal studies were finally published in 2006. By then, Biogen Idec had re-submitted its file to the FDA, and the FDA had once again scheduled a fast-track review. Tysabri received its new approval in June 2006 – only the second time in FDA history that a withdrawn drug was permitted back on the market (the other was Lotronex used to treat irritable bowel syndrome).

How effective is Tysabri?

TYSABRI WAS EVALUATED in two key studies: AFFIRM, which compared the drug to placebo; and SENTINEL, which compared the combination of Tysabri and Avonex with Avonex alone. Both studies used a dose of 300 mg given every four weeks by infusion.

In AFFIRM, the annualized relapse rate was reduced 66% with Tysabri compared to placebo; two-thirds of people taking Tysabri experienced no relapses during the two-year study compared to 41% in the placebo group.[33] The drug also reduced the number of new MRI lesions by over 80% compared to placebo, and a majority of people developed no new lesions while on the drug. These were very impressive results.

The effect of the drug on progression was 40%. Disability progression occurred in 17% of people on Tysabri compared to 29% with placebo. So there was a disconnect between the drug's effect on relapses/MRI and its lesser impact on progression, something that's also been seen with other MS drugs.

Side effects included headache, flushing and skin reactions at the time of infusion, but the drug was generally well tolerated. There was the possibility that people taking Tysabri would develop infections because of the effect of the drug on the immune system, but this didn't appear to be a major problem. A potential concern was the cancer risk: five people on Tysabri developed new cancers (compared to one in the placebo group), and one person who had previously been treated for melanoma (skin cancer) died of melanoma during the study.

The second study was the notorious SENTINEL trial, in which two people developed PML.[34] Although planned as a two-year trial, only one year's worth of data were obtained because the trial was stopped early.

SENTINEL was something of an oddball study. Since some people being considered for Tysabri would already be taking a beta-interferon, the FDA wanted a study that would say something about how the two drugs interacted. It was an attractive notion to Biogen, which manufacturered Avonex. As it turned out, taking the two drugs together did have an effect: the half-life of Tysabri was prolonged by 30% when Avonex was on board.[6] The half-life is the time it takes for one-half of a drug to be cleared from the body, which means the drug is essentially gone after about six half-lives. (So a drug with a half-life of eight hours will take 48 hours to clear. The half-life of Tysabri is 6-

9 days, meaning it takes about seven weeks to be eliminated.) So while PML has generally been attributed to the profound immunosuppression caused by combining two MS drugs, part of the problem may have been that Tysabri persists in the body longer because of the Avonex. That said, the usefulness of a combined Tysabri-Avonex trial was limited: few people in the real world would take the two drugs together, not least because the combined cost would be ruinous (a lesson not learned by the CombiRx trialists, who combined an interferon with Copaxone, to no greater effect).

As it turned out, SENTINEL showed that there was little to recommend the idea of taking the two drugs together. Certainly the combination was more effective than Avonex alone, which hardly needed a study to make the point. In fact, Avonex did especially poorly in this study. The annualized relapse rate with Avonex was almost identical to what was seen with placebo in the AFFIRM study (0.82 vs. 0.81), which may make some wonder about the effectiveness of Avonex. An obvious shortcoming was that the combination wasn't compared to Tysabri alone, so it isn't known if the two drugs together are worth the extra trouble and expense. Such a study is now impossible. With two PML cases in the trial, it was agreed that Tysabri should not be combined with another immune-active drug.[35] (The sole exception has been the GLANCE study, which combined Tysabri with glatiramer acetate.[36] The results suggested that this drug combination was safe, however unlikely it is to be used in real life.)

Taken together, the results of the two Tysabri studies suggested that the drug was more effective than the injectable MS medications – perhaps even twice as effective. This filled a need, which is why the

FDA allowed the drug back onto the market. Subsequent studies have indicated that if a person isn't responding to a first-line treatment (an interferon or Copaxone), they're better off starting Tysabri than switching to another one of the injectables.[37]

The FDA was keen to approve Tysabri but did impose conditions. Tysabri was generally reserved for people who had failed to respond to one of the injectable MS drugs or were unable to tolerate them. The drug monograph also included a black-box warning about the risk of PML. The drug could only be administered by doctors enrolled in a special program (called TOUCH), which required frequent monitoring to detect any new cases of PML. The drug's manufacturer was also required to put a risk management program in place, and to provide periodic updates on the number of PML cases. Safety is also being monitored in an ongoing global observational study called TYGRIS.

What is JCV antibody testing?

PML WAS A VERY DARK CLOUD hanging over Tysabri and it created a great deal of uncertainty about the drug, even among its advocates (of which there were many). One way to cut the perceived risk down to size was to introduce an assay that would test for the presence of JCV to help doctors assess the PML risk. This the manufacturer did, and the Stratify test received FDA approval in January 2012. A new and more accurate test made its appearance a year later.[38] For this test, a blood sample is analysed for the presence of antibodies to JCV. A positive test (i.e. that you have antibodies to the virus) just means that you've been exposed to the virus at some point. It doesn't mean that you have an active infection.

If a person is antibody-positive, the risk of developing PML while on Tysabri is much higher – about 1 in 1000 (0.1%) if there are no other risk factors, 3 per 1000 if you stay on the drug for two years, and about 1 in 77 people (1.3%) if the person has received an immunosuppressant at some point and stays on Tysabri for two years. This doesn't mean that a person who is antibody-positive can't start taking Tysabri, but it might be prudent to explore other options. If Tysabri is started, its use may be limited to two years and another treatment will have to be used to replace it. One concern with stopping Tysabri is that MS symptoms are likely to become more severe, and any subsequent therapies may not be effective at preventing this surge in disease activity. Another concern is the emerging concept that some people who stop Tysabri may have "subclinical PML" (i.e. undetected), which may develop into full-blown PML after they start another treatment.

If a person is antibody-negative, he/she may be considered for Tysabri because the risk of developing PML is probably very low (but not zero). However, this may lend a false sense of security because of the many uncertainties about antibody testing.

The first issue is the rate of false-negative test results, i.e. the test says you're negative but you are actually positive, reported to occur in about 5% of cases.[39] In addition, about 6% will "revert" (i.e. go from positive to negative) in a given year;[40] since this is biologically unlikely (either you've been exposed to the virus or you haven't), it undoubtedly reflects the limits of detection of the assay. So the overall error rate of

JCV antibody testing may be as high as 10% or so. This is a conservative estimate: some studies have indicated that over one in three tests may be wrong.[41]

Secondly, a person's antibody status can change from negative to positive during treatment; this occurs in about 7% of people per year,[40,42] although recent studies have reported that as many as one-third of people will become antibody-positive within a year of starting Tysabri.[43] One reason for this may be that the person was positive all along but the test wasn't sensitive enough to detect the antibodies. Another reason is that Tysabri may affect the immune response to JCV, so that Tysabri exposure itself becomes a risk factor for developing antibodies to the virus. How this might work hasn't been determined. It's known that Tysabri stimulates the release of B cells from bone marrow,[44] and there's some research that suggests that the drug may either promote the entry of the virus into the brain, or may actually increase the likelihood that the virus will reactivate.[45,46] Both possibilities are disturbing scenarios.

Recent efforts have cast the high seroconversion rate (i.e. going from antibody-negative to -positive) in a somewhat different light. Higher amounts of antibody are said to be evidence of greater virus activity, and these people may have a greater risk of developing PML than people with lesser amounts of antibody.[47,48] One could view this as an attempt to recast the JCV story so that merely testing positive for JCV antibodies wouldn't necessarily flag a person as being at high risk of PML. This may make starting Tysabri less of a gamble, but it will be a gamble nevertheless until more is known about the effects of Tysabri on the virus itself.

There may also be individual differences that affect risk. A few studies have found that men are more likely to test JCV antibody-positive.[41,49] A different study reported something a bit contrary: that a majority of PML cases occurred in people weighing 75 kilograms (165 pounds) or less, suggesting that higher drug exposure (i.e. 4 mg of Tysabri per kg of body weight) substantially increases the risk of developing PML.[50] So we return again to the idea that the standard 300 mg dose once a month may be too high for many people.

These issues need further clarification. But because of the uncertainties about JCV antibody testing, it's best to have your antibody status checked every 6-12 months.

Starting treatment with Tysabri

IF YOU AND YOUR DOCTOR decide that Tysabri is the best choice for you, you should have a JCV antibody test before you start treatment. If you are antibody-negative, your chances of developing PML are very low. But you will need periodic blood tests (ideally every 6 months) to ensure that you are still JCV antibody-negative. Some doctors may put off initial antibody testing, arguing that the PML risk is minimal even in antibody-positive people in the first two years of treatment. This is a rather short-sighted approach. Many people may well prefer not to start Tysabri if they know they'll have to come off the drug in a couple of years. An upfront antibody test is preferable so that you have all the information you need for a truly informed decision about treatment.

Tysabri is administered by a slow drip into the vein once a month (although there are studies that suggest that less frequent dosing is just as effective[51,52]). The procedure is usually performed in a specialized infusion centre or hospital. The infusion takes about an hour, but additional time (about an hour) is needed to ensure that you aren't developing a hypersensitivity reaction to the drug; this occurs in less than 1% of people. Typical symptoms of a hypersensitivity reaction include rash, itchy skin, dizziness (especially when standing up), fever, flushing, nausea, chest pain and difficulty breathing.

While on treatment, you will need periodic blood tests to assess your liver function. Liver damage can occur at any time while on Tysabri and the blood test can detect this early. If blood tests aren't done and you develop liver injury, one of the signs is jaundice – an indication that significant damage has occurred (and that Tysabri needs to be stopped).

Other side effects that can occur with Tysabri are headache, fatigue, joint pain, swelling in your hands or feet, depression and diarrhea. Tysabri may also increase your risk of developing an infection. The most common infections are a urinary tract infection, respiratory tract infection (such as pneumonia), gastroenteritis (which feels like stomach flu), tooth infections, tonsillitis, and vaginitis in women.

As a general rule, people tolerate Tysabri fairly well. Many people say that they feel much better on Tysabri compared to when they were on no treatment.[53] But if you do develop any side effects, report them as soon as possible to your doctor or MS nurse.

Can I stop Tysabri?

IF YOU START TYSABRI, you may be counselled to stay on the drug for an indefinite time provided you remain JCV antibody-negative. But be aware that this won't be risk-free: duration of exposure to Tysabri is a risk factor for developing PML even if you don't become JCV antibody-positive. The chances of becoming JCV antibody-positive are about 5-7% per year (and may well be higher).[40,42] Since the PML risk goes up with cumulative exposure to Tysabri, doctors will sometimes recommend changing medications after two or three years whether or not you become antibody-positive – just to be on the safe side. Others will continue the treatment until you become JCV antibody-positive, or continue Tysabri until a problem develops, practices that probably contribute to the rising incidence of PML we've seen.

What this means is that many people won't be able to continue their Tysabri treatment – they'll need to switch to another drug at some point. So what are your options when you stop Tysabri? No treatment isn't advised because of the risk of an MS flare-up after stopping Tysabri (and the need to keep treating your MS). As mentioned previously, opinion is divided on whether this surge in MS symptoms means your MS is going back to the way it was before treatment,[54,55] or is an actual rebound, in which the disease becomes more active and symptoms become worse than they were before.[56-58] Needless to say there is this same risk of increased MS activity if you stop the drug on your own (so deciding to quit "cold turkey" isn't a good plan).

Can you go back the way you came – to one of the first-line injectables? You wouldn't want to re-start a drug that you were on before since we can assume it wasn't working for you or you found the side effects to be unacceptable. As for the other drugs in this category, there have been few studies looking at whether "de-escalating" treatment will work.

What little research there is has shown mixed results. One small study found that people switching from Tysabri to Copaxone didn't have a rebound, and two-thirds had no relapses for a year.[59] Another, even smaller study found that disease activity flared up after switching to Copaxone – in fact, there was no advantage to taking Copaxone compared to a placebo.[60] And in the RESTORE study, after being free of relapses while on Tysabri, most people who switched to Copaxone experience a flare-up in their MS and needed additional treatment.[61]

One approach would be to switch to an oral medication such as Aubagio, Tecfidera or Gilenya. No studies have looked at whether a switch from Tysabri to either Aubagio or Tecfidera is safe and effective; this approach is now being examined in a phase IV study of Aubagio and in the Strategy observational study of Tecfidera. So at the moment the better option may be to switch from Tysabri to Gilenya (see Chapter 8). One study found that there was a flare-up of MS activity, most notably in the first month of switching.[62] This is the in-between period when the effects of Tysabri are wearing off, and the effects of Gilenya haven't fully kicked in yet. Subsequent studies have indicated that the timing of the switch is important.[63,64] The current thinking is that the switch to Gilenya should be made about two months after stopping Tysabri,[64] although some have argued that one month off is enough of a drug holiday before switching to Gilenya.[65]

Of course the drug you switch to will depend on your particular circumstances. Tysabri has remained highly popular among neurologists, despite the drug's potential to cause severe, often fatal side effects. But as more treatment options become available, it's likely that Tysabri will be kept in reserve as the third or fourth drug choice unless a person has very active disease from the outset and is at high risk of progression.

CHAPTER 8

WHAT IS GILENYA?

IN THE EARLY 1980S, A NEW DRUG that suppressed the immune system became an important treatment to prevent tissue rejection in people undergoing an organ transplant. That drug, cyclosporine, was derived from a type of fungus and it sparked interest in what other immune-active medications could be obtained from fungi.

One fungus of particular interest was *Isaria sinclairii* (also known as *Cordyceps*), which attacks and kills insects and which has long been used in Chinese traditional medicine as a fountain of youth – the type of claim that only a traditional remedy could make. Japanese researchers discovered that an extract of *Iscaria* (called ISP-1) was much more potent than cyclosporine,[1] and it became the lead compound for a new line of research. This led to the discovery in 1992 of FTY720,[2] named after researcher Tetsuro Fujita, the Taito company (now Mitsui Seito), and Yoshitomi Pharmaceuticals (now Mitsubishi Tanabe Pharma).[3]

FTY720 was initially investigated as an anti-rejection drug, but it was also studied as a possible treatment for various autoimmune disorders, such as Type 1 diabetes and lupus.[4,5] The main plan was to have a drug that could be used in conjunction with cyclosporine, which attracted the attention of Sandoz (now Novartis), the Swiss manufacturer of cyclosporine. A decade later, FTY720 was renamed fingolimod, acquiring the trade name of Gilenya when the drug was approved for the treatment of MS in 2010.

Throughout its development, Gilenya was in competition with cladribine to become the first oral treatment for MS. Cladribine won that race, but was soon withdrawn due to safety concerns (but may yet return). That left Gilenya as the first oral drug to achieve widespread use as a treatment for MS.

How does Gilenya work?

CONVENTIONAL IMMUNOSUPPRESSANT DRUGS typically work by destroying immune cells. But early in the development of Gilenya, it became apparent that the drug acted very differently. It did reduce the number of immune cells (such as T cells) circulating in the body, but not by killing them off.

Lymphocytes, such as T cells and B cells, normally move throughout the blood and lymphatic systems, patrolling the body as part of their routine surveillance. During their travels, T cells regularly visit the lymphoid organs (such as the lymph nodes and the spleen), with homing signals acting like a GPS, enabling them to find these pit stops. While inside the lymphoid organs, immune cells share what they've found – bits and pieces of antigens that they've collected in their travels. If one of these antigens indicates there's a problem somewhere in the body, the T cells quickly expand their population, leave the lymphoid organ and go off in search of trouble (where there is infection, inflammation or tissue damage).

This movement of lymphocytes in and out of the lymphoid organs has to be regulated to prevent traffic jams. One of the traffic cops is called S1P (for sphingosine-1-phosphate), a signalling molecule that gives activated T cells the green light to leave the lymph node.

This is where Gilenya comes in. Once inside the body, Gilenya undergoes a chemical change (called phosphorylation) so that it resembles S1P. This bit of mimicry initially stimulates the S1P receptor on T cells (called an agonist effect). But shortly thereafter, the receptors are taken off-line (a functional antagonist effect),[6,7] akin to someone unplugging the TV because the volume is too loud. With S1P receptors out of commission, T cells don't get the message to leave the lymph node. This effect is quite selective (B cells are still able to get out[8]). The main T cells affected are central memory T cells (TCMs), which are highly active in MS.[9,10] Another type of T cell, called effector memory T cells (TEMs), typically lack the GPS (called CCR7), don't go into the lymph nodes in the first place, and so they can continue to patrol for infection.

In practical terms, what this means is that soon after taking Gilenya, the pool of activated T cells available to invade the central nervous system is reduced substantially. The total population of lymphocytes doesn't appear to be affected;[11] rather, the distribution is changed, with some locked up in the lymph nodes and others circulating throughout the body. Within two weeks of starting fingolimod at the usual dose (0.5 mg per day), the number of activated

T cells detectable in the blood stream is reduced by about 70%.[12] The number of T cells remains at this low level during treatment, but does return to normal within a few months of stopping the drug as the trapped T cells re-emerge into the circulation.[12]

How effective is Gilenya in relapsing-remitting MS?

THE FIRST STUDY OF GILENYA in RRMS was a phase II trial published in 2006.[13] A total of 281 participants received one of two doses of fingolimod (1.25 or 5.0 mg per day) or a placebo for six months. The study showed that Gilenya reduced the relapse rate by 55% compared to placebo and was effective in reducing the number of inflammatory lesions seen on MRI. The study was later extended to two years, during which everyone in the placebo group was switched to Gilenya.[14] Among those completing two years on treatment (about two-thirds of those in the original study), 77% experienced no new relapses and 79-91% had no inflammatory lesions on their MRI.

So Gilenya did appear to be very effective in MS. But one problem was the dose (as we've seen before with Tysabri). The minimum effective dose is usually determined in a dose-ranging study, which tests different amounts of drug to find the optimal balance between effectiveness and side effects. This was done when fingolimod was being tested as a drug to prevent organ rejection, but not in people with MS. An early safety study tried using a dose of 1 mg per day.[15] A dose-ranging study in people undergoing a kidney transplant found that the highest dose tested (2.5 mg) appeared to be the best.[16] However, subsequent studies began to use a maximum dose of 5 mg per day,[17] although there was early evidence that side effects might be a problem with such a high dose.[18] What appears to have decided the issue was a study that showed that the maximal effect of the drug on lymphocytes occurred with a dose of 5 mg[19] – although it's important to keep in mind that this was still when Gilenya was being investigated as an anti-rejection drug and not for MS.

The lack of a dose-ranging study was a serious shortcoming of the early development program in MS. And in fact, the 5-mg dose was dropped during the second year of the phase II study. Lower doses (1.25 and 0.5 mg) would be used in the phase III studies, with the approved dose (0.5 mg/day) being one-tenth of the dose originally tested – which is unusual to say the least.

The first two phase III studies of Gilenya were called FREEDOMS (for FTY720 Research Evaluating Effects of Daily Oral Therapy in Multiple Sclerosis), which was a two-year study;[20] and TRANSFORMS (Trial Assessing Injectable Interferon versus FTY720 Oral in Relapsing–Remitting Multiple Sclerosis), which was a one-year study.[21] These were very large trials, together enrolling over 2,500 people. Both studied two doses of Gilenya (0.5 mg and 1.25 per day). FREEDOMS compared the drug to a placebo, while TRANSFORMS compared the drug to weekly Avonex.

Overall, both of these studies showed that Gilenya was highly effective in RRMS. The annualized relapse rate (ARR) with the 0.5 mg dose of Gilenya was 0.18 in FREEDOMS, and 0.16 in TRANSFORMS. By comparison, the ARR was 0.40 with placebo and 0.33 with Avonex, respectively. This represented a 52-54% reduction in the relapse rate with Gilenya, all the more impressive since one of these comparisons was against an active drug. Indeed, the relapse rate among people taking a placebo was very similar to what was seen for people taking Avonex. (As you'll recall, Avonex also performed much like a placebo in the SENTINEL trial of Tysabri.) Both of these studies also showed that Gilenya was highly effective in reducing disease activity in the brain as seen on MRI, and there were also modest effects (about 30% compared to placebo) on disability progression. The higher 1.25-mg dose didn't appear to add much benefit, so it was dropped and the 0.5-mg dose was the one that would later be approved.

A third phase III study, FREEDOMS II appeared to confirm what had already been seen before.[22] ARR was 0.21 among people on Gilenya and 0.40 for those on placebo (a 48% reduction in relapses). The effect on disability progression was disappointing – 17% lower with Gilenya compared to placebo, and this difference wasn't significant.

Two analyses later sifted through various studies and both concluded that Gilenya was substantially better at reducing relapses compared to a first-line interferon or Copaxone.[23,24] But while it's generally believed that Gilenya is more potent than the injectables (only Avonex has been used in a direct comparison), this can only be determined for certain with head-to-head studies.

What are the possible side effects of Gilenya?

THE MOST COMMON SIDE EFFECT with Gilenya in the FREEDOMS and TRANSFORMS trials was infections, although the overall risk was similar to what was seen with placebo or Avonex.[20,21] Closer examination showed that there was a higher risk of bronchitis, which occurred in 8% of people (compared to 3.6% with placebo). Also more common were herpes infections in FREEDOMS, although in TRANSFORMS the rate of herpes infections was slightly lower with Gilenya compared to Avonex. But herpes was a serious concern: two people died in TRANSFORMS because of herpes infections. The first person hadn't had chickenpox (varicella zoster virus [VZV], one of the herpesviruses) as a child, contracted the disease while on Gilenya and a course of steroids, and was unable to fight off the infection. In the second case, the person developed a herpes-related brain infection, received a course of steroids (further suppressing the immune response) and died two months later. These tragic events led to the requirement that people be tested to ensure that they have already had chickenpox; if they have had no prior exposure, VZV vaccination is recommended. It may be prudent for everyone thinking of starting Gilenya to get vaccinated beforehand.

Blood tests found that 7-16% showed elevated liver enzymes during Gilenya treatment, so liver function needs to be checked before starting the drug, every three months for the first year, and periodically thereafter.

An unusual effect was swelling of part of the eye (called macular edema). Gilenya can cause leakage of the blood vessels in the eye,[25] which leads to swelling in the eye and vision problems. There were seven cases (0.8%) in FREEDOMS, and six cases (0.7%) in TRANSFORMS, with most occurring with the higher dose. A slightly lower rate (0.4%) was reported in the extension of the FREEDOMS

II trial.[26] To guard against this possible complication, an eye test is needed 3-4 months after starting Gilenya, although macular edema can develop over a year afterward. If macular edema does develop, the problem generally goes away when treatment is stopped. It isn't known if the risk of macular edema is higher in people who have a higher risk of eye problems, such as those with diabetes. Since macular edema may be difficult to distinguish from the vision problems that can occur with MS, it's important to report any eye symptoms to your doctor.

A potential concern with many immune-active drugs is cancer risk, because one of the functions of the immune system is to patrol the body in search of abnormal cells, including cancer cells.[27] Gilenya's effects on immune cells (T and B cells) means there's a theoretical possibility that it could impair immunosurveillance,[28] so this issue was investigated in the clinical trials. In FREEDOMS there were eight cancers in the Gilenya groups (an incidence of 0.9%) compared to 10 in the placebo group (2.3%).[20] In FREEDOMS II, the incidence of a type of skin cancer was 3% with Gilenya 0.5 mg compared to 1% with placebo.[22] In TRANSFORMS, there were 12 cancers in the Gilenya groups (1.4%) compared to one cancer (0.2%) with Avonex.[21] So it's possible that there's a slightly increased risk of cancers with Gilenya, although the actual risk won't be known until people have been on the drug longer. It may be that if there is a higher risk, it's only for some types of cancers. So it may be a good idea to be checked annually for skin cancers (even if you're not taking Gilenya). However, cancer risk is probably not a great concern. S1P signalling has been implicated in the spread of cancer, and Gilenya and other S1P blocking drugs are now being studied as possible anti-cancer drugs for certain types of cancer, such as breast, ovarian and prostate cancer.[29-31]

In looking at the side-effect profile of Gilenya, what distinguished the drug – and was the greatest cause for concern – was its effects on the heart. Gilenya targets four S1P receptors (designated 1, 3, 4 and 5), and these can be found throughout the body. So the drug's interaction with S1P receptors isn't restricted to blood cells. It will also affect these receptors wherever else they're found, resulting in side effects. This is a common situation with receptor-targeting drugs because of the body's sense of economy: it uses the same receptors, substances and biochemical pathways for multiple functions, so targeting one thing will also affect other things. For example, targeting the neurotransmitter acetylcholine is useful to treat urinary incontinence (with drugs such as Ditropan [oxybutynin] or Detrol [tolterodine]), but will also cause dry mouth and blurred vision.

So when Gilenya is first started, it will interact with S1P receptors in the heart and blood vessels, which can result in three heart-related effects. The first is an initial slowing of the heart rate (your pulse). This is because when you start Gilenya, the drug has an initial stimulatory (agonist) effect on the receptors that normally slow down the heart.[32] In most people, this heart rate decrease (called bradycardia) amounts to about 8-15 beats per minute.[33,34] Heart rate may be further slowed if Gilenya is taken with some blood pressure medications that slow heart rate, such as beta-blockers.[35] In the Gilenya trials, the heart rate was reduced about 8 beats per minute on average,[36] so if your normal resting heart rate was 75 beats per minute, it might go down to 60-67 beats per minute. This effect appears to be time-limited. As your body gets used to the drug, S1P receptors are taken off-line (the functional antagonist effect previously mentioned) and the heart rate goes back to normal. A slower heart rate is most apparent in the first day of dosing, reaching its lowest point about 4-5 hours after taking the first dose of the drug before it begins to recover. Heart rate typically returns to normal within a week or so.[33,36] Usually there aren't any symptoms associated with a slowed heart rate, but some people may experience dizziness, chest pain or palpitations. The simplest solution is to get up and walk about during the first dose, which stimulates the heart to beat a little faster.

In some cases, a slowing of the heart rate may also be associated with an effect on the electrical signalling in the heart, as seen on an electrocardiogram (ECG). This can result in abnormalities such as heart block, an interruption in the normal electrical signalling. This can occur in normal individuals, even younger people and athletes, but is only detected when the person is hooked up to an ECG machine. But in more severe cases, such as in people with heart disease, heart block can lead to a heart attack or sudden death.

Because of its effects on heart cells, Gilenya has the potential to disturb the normal heart rhythm. In the FREEDOMS and TRANSFORMS trials, about 1% of people taking Gilenya experienced heart block.[20,21] In the observational FIRST study, the rate was higher – about 2%.[37] The heart block seen with Gilenya usually isn't associated with any symptoms or long-term consequences, and no treatment is typically needed. In some cases, people are kept overnight in hospital and closely monitored to ensure that their heart rhythm returns to normal.

The third heart-related effect is blood pressure changes, resulting in a slightly lower (hypotension) or higher (hypertension) blood pressure. During longer-term use, there appears to be a small increase in blood pressure of about 3-5 mmHg.[38] So if your usual blood pressure was 120/80 (systolic 120 mmHg, diastolic 80 mmHg), it might settle in somewhere around 125/85, which is still considered to be within the normal range. However, sustained hypertension may be more of a concern in older people with other cardiovascular risk factors (e.g. diabetes, smoking, obesity, high cholesterol, etc.).

The effects of Gilenya on heart conduction were the most important. They appeared to be fairly uncommon, typically resolved within the first month of treatment and didn't seem especially serious. The risk appeared to be highest in the first few hours after taking the first dose, so the FDA required a six-hour observation period for anyone starting Gilenya.

Safety concerns were raised about a year after the drug was approved by the FDA, in what seemed to some as a replay of the Tysabri story. In November 2011, one person was reported to have died within a day of taking Gilenya. The person had heart disease as well as MS and was taking two heart medications at the time of death. The FDA investigated and a month later reported that it couldn't determine if the death was caused by Gilenya or not.[39] Then in May 2012, the FDA issued a second report on people who had died while on Gilenya. During the eight years that Gilenya had been in development and on the market, 30,000 people had been exposed to the drug and 31 had died (so about 1 per 1000).[40] While this mortality rate was in line with what's seen in the general population, some of these deaths were heart-related and there were lingering questions about the person who died within a day of starting treatment. But in a subsequent communiqué, and in an update in December 2012, the FDA stated that it couldn't definitively conclude that Gilenya was a contributing factor in any of these deaths.[39,41]

The European Medicines Agency (the European equivalent of the FDA) looked into this issue as well. What the EMA wanted to investigate were four heart-related deaths and two cases of people who died in their sleep. In its April 2012 report, the EMA found that most of the deaths occurred in people with heart disease or who were taking other medications as well, so it couldn't determine whether or not Gilenya was the actual cause of death.[42] It concluded that with closer monitoring during the first dose, the benefits of Gilenya outweighed the risks of heart problems.

But a new note of caution appeared in revisions to the product label in different countries. In the U.S., two important changes were made. Hourly pulse and blood pressure readings were recommended during the initial six-hour observation period, and an ECG was advised before and after the first dose. Overnight monitoring in hospital was required if people seemed to be running into trouble, or if they had a recent history of severe heart disease (heart attack, angina, stroke, heart failure) or were taking certain heart medications.[43]

Similar monitoring requirements were instituted in other countries, such as Canada.[44] In contrast to the first-line indication in the U.S., Canada approved Gilenya as a second-line drug for use in people who had not done well on an injectable, either because of a lack of effectiveness or side effects. This means that Canadians are generally a bit older when they start taking Gilenya. But the risk of potentially serious heart block (about 1 in a thousand) in Canada is similar to what's seen in other countries.[45]

The need for a six-hour observation period when taking the first dose was a nuisance, and concerns about possible cardiac effects made Gilenya less attractive to some. Gilenya remained on the Top 100 list of drugs in the U.S.,[46] ahead of Betaseron but lagging behind the other injectables, and sales hit a plateau in the months following the label change.[47] That appears to be changing somewhat as doctors become more familiar with Gilenya, monitor them more closely, and are better able to select the best candidates for Gilenya.[48]

The potential safety issues seen with Gilenya and Tysabri ushered in a new phase in MS therapies. The need to weigh the benefits and risks of treatment is now the neurologist's mantra with second-generation MS treatments. It may be that Gilenya and Tysabri will be better able to prevent long-term disability (more time is needed before that will be known for sure), but the price of that effectiveness will be a certain amount of risk.

The first-generation injectables were a low benefit/low risk approach. Some of the newer drugs (e.g. Aubagio) are continuing this strategy. But other therapies are pursuing a more aggressive line – a trend that began with Tysabri and Gilenya and which culminates in Lemtrada, perhaps the most potent of the drugs now available. We'll look at how to assess the benefits and risks of treatment in the final chapter.

What other Gilenya studies are being done?

THE HEART EFFECTS SEEN with Gilenya were known from the very beginning, resulting in much discussion at the FDA between 2005 and the drug's approval in 2010.[49] Two results of this back-and-forth were the decision to discontinue the 1.25-mg dose, and a trial to determine if a lower dose (0.25 mg) might be effective. It's tempting to speculate that had low-dose Gilenya been tested sooner, we might well have avoided many of the cardiac effects (as well as the need for a six-hour observation period) that can occur when starting the drug. Unfortunately, the results of this lower-dose study, which will compare two doses of Gilenya (0.5 and 0.25 mg) with Copaxone, aren't expected for a few years.

Current studies of Gilenya are investigating two key ideas – one theoretical and one practical. Unlike many MS drugs, Gilenya actually enters the CNS,[50] and it may have some important effects there. Experimental studies have suggested that Gilenya has beneficial effects in the brain, improving survival of the cells that produce myelin (oligodendrocytes) and promoting remyelination of damaged nerve fibres.[51-54] It remains to be seen if these effects will produce any benefits during the long-term course of MS. But the possibility of preserving nerve fibres has prompted some preliminary research into Gilenya as a treatment for spinal cord injury or for people who have suffered a stroke.[55,56]

The best practical test of the possible neuroprotective effect of Gilenya is the INFORMS trial, which is studying the effectiveness of the drug in primary-progressive MS. The thinking was that the anti-inflammatory effects of Gilenya were unlikely to have much impact on the neurodegeneration seen in PPMS, so if there was a benefit, it could be due to the drug's direct effects on the brain. Unfortunately, the early word is that INFORMS failed to show a benefit.[57] This raises three immediate possibilities: either PPMS is somehow different than RRMS in its underlying disease process (which hasn't been established); treatment was started too late; or whatever effects Gilenya has on cells in the brain are insufficient to provide a benefit. More will be known when the full results of the study are presented.

ANOTHER AVENUE OF RESEARCH is also worth mentioning. With the broad range of therapies now available, there is now the issue of determining the optimal sequence of medications. While we'll look at this issue in more detail in the last chapter, some studies have looked at whether Gilenya is an option in people who can no longer take Tysabri. (No studies have looked at the best option for people who don't respond to Gilenya.)

The main challenge is that when you stop Tysabri, there's a very real risk that MS will flare up again. A few small studies found that a majority of people who switched from Tysabri to Gilenya had a relapse.[58-60] Much of the problem seemed to occur during the initial three-month switchover period as Tysabri was eliminated from the body and Gilenya wasn't fully effective yet. A German switch study found that most relapses occurred in the first eight weeks of stopping Tysabri.[61] While many people (42%) had a relapse after starting Gilenya, considerably more (70%) relapsed if they stopped Tysabri and didn't start another treatment, so there was a treatment effect with

Gilenya. Once the drug takes effect, the risk of relapses appears to go down. In the FIRST study, 17% of people coming off Tysabri had a relapse in the first month, but this went down to 6% in the second month, and less than 2% in the fourth month.[62]

People coming off Tysabri will generally need something potent to regain control of MS inflammation, so Gilenya appears to be a good option. As mentioned in the previous chapter, it isn't known if other oral drugs will be effective in this situation. It will need to be established if a more potent drug, such as Lemtrada, is a safe alternative after someone has been taking Tysabri. One potential concern is that subclinical PML may develop into PML after Tysabri is stopped and another immune-active drug is started. For example, PML has developed in about a dozen cases of people who switched from Tysabri to Gilenya.[63] Until recently, the thinking was that PML began during Tysabri but no symptoms were apparent, and no one detected it until after Gilenya was started. That view may change now that one PML case has now been reported in someone on Gilenya with no prior exposure to Tysabri (there had been prior exposure to Rebif).[64] The person had been taking Gilenya for just over four years, so the current thinking is that prolonged immune suppression contributed to the development of PML. It isn't known if a non-specific immune suppression is sufficient on its own, if there is something unique to Gilenya's effects on the body that resulted in PML. For example, Gilenya is known to impair the body's ability to suppress viruses – as evidenced by the two deaths due to herpes infections in the TRANSFORMS trial, and by the viral reactivation (such as shingles) that can occur during treatment. But this will require further study. But to put things into perspective, there has been only one clear-cut case of PML that appears to be attributable to Gilenya among the 100,000 people who have taken the drug. So the risk of PML with Gilenya appears to be very small indeed.

A more worrisome prospect is that PML can emerge after prolonged immune suppression, which raises the theoretical possibility of it developing with many drugs in the MS arsenal. It may also be that people with MS are uniquely susceptible to PML because of an altered response to viral infections, which people have speculated about for decades. More research will need to be done to clarify why PML develops in people with MS.

Despite some concerns about safety, Gilenya remains an important option for people who need a more potent drug to control their MS. In terms of effectiveness, it appears to be sandwiched between Tecfidera and Tysabri – a little more potent than Tecfidera, a little less than Tysabri – although only head-to-head studies will determine this for sure. It's a good option for people who prefer an oral over an injection or infusion drug; those who haven't responded well enough to a prior therapy; and people with highly active MS who aren't good candidates for Tysabri because of exposure to the JC virus.

CHAPTER 9

WHAT IS TECFIDERA?

ONE OF THE NEWEST MS TREATMENTS is Tecfidera (dimethyl fumarate; BG-12), although its history makes it the oldest of the new therapies. As we've seen with other MS drugs, the origins of Tecfidera were based on a largely mistaken idea, but they may have also owed a little something to homeopathic medicine.

In 1959, a German chemist named Schweckendiek, who suffered from psoriasis (an autoimmune skin disorder), thought that a mixture of fumaric acid derivatives (FAD) might help his condition.[1] Fumaric acid is a fruity-tasting, naturally occurring compound found in certain mushrooms, lichen and moss. The chemical is also produced by the skin – hence its connection with psoriasis – and can be found in urine.[2]

What was appealing to a chemist was that fumarate is a step in the Krebs cycle, an important series of biochemical reactions by which cells produce energy. The steps involved in this process were worked out by a German physician, Hans Adolf Krebs, who had received a Nobel Prize just a few years before Schweckendiek's FAD experiment, so perhaps the Krebs cycle was top-of-mind. Schweckendiek believed that psoriasis cells were lacking energy, so he reasoned that supplying more fumarate might correct this deficiency. His solution was to ingest FADs, bathe in a FAD solution and apply some of it to his skin.

Applying fumarates to the skin would seem to be counterintuitive because these chemicals can cause nasty skin lesions. But the underlying idea may have owed something to early medical concepts that crop up in homeopathic medicine: the Law of Similars, which supposes that an effective drug will cause symptoms similar to the ones it's trying to treat; and the notion that the only difference between a poison and a medicine is the dose. In homeopathy, diluting the substance is believed to weaken a drug's poisonous effects while preserving its usefulness as a therapy.

Schweckendiek's self-treatment did improve his psoriasis, and in this he was fortunate. The treatment plan was then modified to a combination of a healthy diet, oral FAD and a FAD ointment or bathing oil.[3] This appeared to be a successful regimen for some people with psoriasis, and is the reason for the oft-repeated claim that fumarates have been in use for the past 50 years. However, this isn't strictly correct. Fumarates had a very mixed track record in psoriasis and their use was limited by word-of-mouth. The opinion among many German dermatologists was that fumarates could cause some unpleasant side effects and so they were largely abandoned as a treatment option.[3] In the 1980s – some 25 years later – dermatologists still considered fumaric acid to be "far too toxic for clinical use" and warned that it should not be used as a psoriasis drug.[4]

FADs were given a second look in the late 1980s. The full regimen of ointments and baths was dropped and just the oral drug was investigated. This was prudent because fumarates were notorious for being highly irritating to the skin and could cause severe skin rashes in people who were sensitive to them[5] – which presumably didn't include Schweckendiek marinating in his chemical bath. But this problem of skin irritation would re-emerge a decade later.

A mixture of FADs was administered orally in a small study of 13 people and about one-half showed a significant improvement, although four people had to stop therapy because of severe stomach pain.[6] By mere coincidence, one of the researchers was named Krebs.

These preliminary results were encouraging enough to prompt larger studies. The first was performed in the Netherlands and reported the same result – a significant improvement in about 50% of people.[7] The study used enteric-coated tablets but stomach pain and diarrhea were still common problems, so the treatment was still considered to be experimental. Subsequent studies also found that fumaric acid therapy was often highly effective for psoriasis, although some people found that their skin lesions got worse and many complained of gastrointestinal upset and flushing.[8-10] As a result, the course of treatment was generally limited to a few weeks or months.[11]

But these results were good enough to generate enthusiasm for one formulation of FAD, called Fumaderm, manufactured by the German firm Fumaderm AG and distributed by Fumedica. The drug was approved in Germany for the treatment of psoriasis in 1994. Fumaderm would become the most widely prescribed oral medication for psoriasis in Germany, although the drug wasn't marketed in most of Europe or in North America.

Fumaderm was an assortment of fumaric acid compounds but one of these – dimethyl fumarate (DMF) – appeared to be the main active ingredient. So DMF became the focus of research and was investigated as a treatment for various things – including cancer, to prevent organ rejection following transplantation, and as a cure for baldness.[12-14] A new preparation, called BG-00012 , was developed, ostensibly as a second-generation Fumaderm although it was simply a reformulation rather than a new and improved compound. Other fumaric acid derivatives were removed so that only DMF remained. This stripped-down version of the formula would later bear the stripped-down name of BG-12. Its Fumaderm moniker, FAG-201, was shelved.

DMF was shown to have potent effects on the immune system, driving activated T cells to self-destruct (called apoptosis),[15] which suggested that a promising avenue of research for BG-12 might be for autoimmune disorders such as MS. This attracted the attention of Biogen, the manufacturers of Avonex and Tysabri, which licensed the worldwide rights (excluding Germany) for the development of the drug in September 2003.[16] Biogen (soon to be Biogen Idec) and Fumaderm AG held hands for three years until a phase II study of BG-12 was completed. One day after the results were announced, Biogen Idec tied the knot with Fumaderm AG,[17] securing its hold on BG-12 and paving the way for developing the drug as a new treatment for MS. Phase III studies of BG-12 were completed in psoriasis, but Biogen

Idec opted not to pursue this indication any further,[18] presumably so the company could focus all of its efforts on MS.

BG-12 quickly paid dividends. With the brand name of Tecfidera, the drug was approved by the FDA for the treatment of relapsing MS in March 2013 – and earned almost one billion dollars in sales by the close of the year.

How does Tecfidera work?

AS WE CAN SEE from this brief history, how fumarates work in the treatment of autoimmune disorders isn't entirely clear. Even the Tecfidera product monograph states that the drug's mode of action is unknown.[19] So precisely what Tecfidera does in the body and how it works in MS are ripe for speculation, and many ideas have been floated over the years.

The initial idea – that fumarates re-fuel the Krebs cycle and supply cells with more energy – was a bit nutty and has been largely abandoned. Another suggestion was that Tecfidera shifts the response of inflammatory T cells (Th1 cells) to a less inflammatory (Th2) profile[20] – which is one of the ways that Copaxone and the interferons are said to work. But this is a sort of catch-all answer that doesn't explain much.

One source of confusion is what the active drug is. DMF is considered the active molecule and this is the chemical that's often tested in the lab to identify its effects. Normally a drug has a number of interactions in the body before it is broken down (metabolized) and eliminated, but this isn't the case with DMF. DMF is highly resistant to acids, so it passes through the stomach unchanged. Once DMF reaches the less acidic environment of the small intestine, it's very quickly metabolized (in about two hours).[21] But even before then, as DMF is absorbed, it only lasts about six minutes in the bloodstream before it's broken down by white blood cells. This is so short a time that it's unlikely that DMF has a direct effect on cells, Th1/Th2 or otherwise. In fact, a study of Fumaderm in healthy people found that DMF was not detectable in any of the blood samples that were taken.[22] However, DMF may have indirect effects, as we'll see later.

Since DMF doesn't survive very long in the body, it's important to look at its metabolites (i.e. what's left after it has been broken down). A metabolite of DMF is MMF (monomethyl fumarate), which is also biologically active, so this is probably where we should direct our attention. This distinction between DMF and MMF is important because these two chemicals act somewhat differently. For example, one suggestion was that DMF works in MS by interacting with adhesion molecules of the blood-brain barrier, in effect making them less "sticky".[23,24] This is how Tysabri works in MS, preventing activated T cells from crossing the blood-brain barrier and causing inflammation in the central nervous system (see Chapter 6). DMF may have this effect; its metabolite, MMF, does not.[23] So this method of action is unlikely to be important.

There is some evidence to suggest that MMF can impair the expression of inflammatory Th1 cells;[25] although there are also data suggesting that it doesn't affect Th1 cells but rather stimulates Th2 production[26] (although some have argued against this as well).[27] It may also be that MMF is toxic to lymphocytes and simply reduces the number of activated T cells[28] – which will be important when we look later on at side effects.

In recent years, Tecfidera studies have focused on two separate but inter-related transcription factors (called Nrf-2 and NF-kappaB) that are involved in how the body defends itself against toxic substances. Transcription factors are proteins in cells that enable the body to respond to changing circumstances. These factors function as an On switch. Once activated, they travel to the nucleus, plug into the DNA and cause genes to produce the proteins that are needed (such as enzymes, signalling molecules and so on).

One thing that can trigger transcription factors is reactive oxygen species (ROS, commonly known as "free radicals"). As the term implies, these are oxygen-containing molecules that are highly reactive with molecules in the body. An example is hydrogen peroxide, a powerful oxidant that is used as a bleach (as in peroxide blonde). ROS are produced as a by-product of the body's normal metabolism.

Like many things in the body, ROS can be beneficial or harmful. During infection, the innate immune system uses bursts of ROS like a type of poison gas to kill invading bacteria and viruses. ROS also act as signalling molecules for the immune system, and they are needed during the initial activation of T cells.[29] But excessive ROS can also inhibit T cells and drive them to self-destruct.[30] In the brain, ROS produced by activated immune cells can directly damage nerve cells, the myelin that protects them, and the cells (oligodendrocytes) that produce myelin.[31,32]

If the body can't detoxify the ROS being produced, ROS will accumulate and cause damage to cells (including damage to DNA). So one method is for the blood-brain barrier to actively pump ROS out of the brain. Another approach is for the body to have an antioxidant response to these oxidants. This is one reason why you'll often hear people promoting the benefits of antioxidants such as vitamins C and E.

A chemical such as Tecfidera appears to stimulate the body's antioxidant responses. One way it appears to do this is by inducing the expression of the transcription factor called Nrf-2 (for nuclear factor [erythroid-derived 2]-related factor 2). But just to clarify the expression "inducing an antioxidant response", Tecfidera isn't an anti-oxidant exactly. Perhaps a better description would be that the body perceives the drug as a stressor and defends itself by turning on its antioxidant machinery.

One of the body's lines of defence against oxidative stress is glutathione. In the short term, DMF (but not MMF) appears to deplete cells' stores of glutathione.[33,34] Because this compromises the body's defence mechanisms, the body tries to compensate by turning on Nrf-2, which in turn gears up production of glutathione – resulting in a net gain of glutathione. Both DMF and MMF also appear to directly increase Nrf-2, which may protect sensitive cells (which may include cells in the CNS) from oxidative damage.[35]

Glutathione production also appears to stimulate the production of a key enzyme (called heme oxygenase 1). The main role of this enzyme is to break down dead blood cells (it's the reason that bruises change colour) but it also has anti-inflammatory effects,[27] which may benefit cells in the brain. However, this requires prolonged drug exposure and it isn't clear if DMF or MMF acts long enough for this to have much of an impact.[36]

In opposition to the Nrf-2 pathway is the NF-kappaB pathway. Like Nrf-2, NF-kappaB is a transcription factor but the genes it turns on drive cell division. As part of the immune response, pattern-recognition receptors identify suspicious "profiles" (such as bacteria) and activate NF-kappaB, which then stimulates T cell proliferation and inflammation to combat the infection. This switch can get locked in the On position, so anti NF-kappaB strategies are now the focus of cancer research. The hope is that turning off the switch will stop NF-kappa-B from promoting uncontrolled growth of tumour cells. As a side note, a number of studies have indicated that green tea (or its active compound epigallocatechin-3-gallate [EGCG]) has beneficial effects by suppressing the NF-kappaB switch.[37]

DMF (but not its metabolite) has been shown to inhibit NF-kappaB,[37,39] so this may be one way that DMF induces inflammatory T cells to self-destruct rather than proliferate. There is some evidence that NF-kappaB and Nrf-2 share some cross-talk, although it's too early to hear clearly what they are saying to each other. Increased production of glutathione by Nrf-2 may reduce NF-kappaB; and conversely, NF-kappaB may inactivate Nrf-2.[40]

These speculations about how Tecfidera works are a bit after the fact, in part because the drug belongs to an era when doctors tried out various notions and potions and the more successful therapies earned a place in the doctor's bag. That's one of the reasons that three decades passed from the first recorded instance of fumarates being used in psoriasis and the first scientific trial. In the same vein, researchers are still working out what Aspirin does. This situation isn't dissimilar from the story of interferons and Copaxone: after 20 years of use, we still don't know exactly what they do in MS. But it's very different from the story of Tysabri or Gilenya, which were developed because of their known effects on the immune system.

The effects of Tecfidera on the body's antioxidant defences are the prevailing theory at the moment, but this may change somewhat as more research is done. What is undoubtedly more important for most people is how effective Tecfidera is in MS.

How effective is Tecfidera in relapsing-remitting MS?

BEFORE TECFIDERA WAS DEVELOPED, Fumaderm was examined in a pilot study of 10 people with relapsing-remitting MS in Germany.[41] People received a higher dose (720 mg per day) for 18 weeks, got a one-month break from treatment, then resumed Fumaderm at a lower dose (360 mg per day) for another 48 weeks. The most common side effects were gastrointestinal problems and flushing. These were reportedly mild, although three people (30%) were withdrawn from the trial because of side effects or because they had stopped taking the drug. During the initial higher-dose phase, there were improvements in the number and size of inflammatory lesions seen on MRI, and this effect was maintained during the lower-dose period.

Fumaderm wasn't studied any further in MS. After the pilot study was completed, DMF – ostensibly the less toxic alternative – was ready to go and the phase II trial started recruiting subjects in

November 2004. Biogen was riding high: the DMF trial started in the same month that Tysabri received FDA approval. As things turned out, by the time the DMF trial finished recruiting in March 2005, Tysabri had been withdrawn from the market. We can imagine that fingers were crossed at Biogen during the six months of the DMF study.

The phase II study used different doses to determine the right balance of effectiveness and safety.[42] A total of 256 people with RRMS received a placebo or one of three doses of DMF: either 120 mg once a day, 120 mg three times a day, or 240 mg three times a day. (The dose that was later approved – 240 mg twice-daily – wasn't examined.) About 20% of people withdrew from the study or stopped taking the drug within the initial six months, either because of side effects or for other reasons.

As in the pilot study, the main thing that was looked at was the effect of the drug on MRI lesions. There wasn't much of an impact with the two lower doses (120 mg once or three times per day), indicating that these doses were too low to be effective. For the higher dose group, there was a substantial effect (69% reduction compared to placebo) on the number of new inflammatory lesions.

The effect on relapses was less impressive. In fact, people taking DMF 120 three times per day had a higher relapse rate than those taking a placebo. With the high-dose regimen, the relapse rate was reduced 32% compared to placebo – similar to what is seen with Rebif, Betaseron or Copaxone. The annualized relapse rate (ARR) with the highest dose of DMF was 0.44, which was very high for an MS study conducted in the mid-2000s (substantially higher than the ARR in trials of Gilenya, Aubagio and Lemtrada). This was a bit disappointing. The ARR did go down some more during a second 24-week safety extension so that it was 0.28 at the end of 48 weeks, but this was still a little underwhelming. Overall, 77% of people had no relapses during the 48 weeks of the study and the remainder continued to have relapses.

Gastrointestinal side effects, such as nausea/vomiting, diarrhea and stomach pain, were increasingly common as the dose was increased; 41% of people in the high-dose group experienced at least one of these problems. The most common side effect was flushing, which occurred in almost one-half of the people in the high-dose group. Serious side effects were uncommon. There were some minor effects on the liver, and no significant changes to blood cell counts, so this suggested a good overall safety picture.

These results were very promising, but there are few silver linings without a cloud. While the trial was running, DMF was implicated in what became known as the Chinese sofa scandal. In 2007, there was an epidemic of severe skin rashes in Finland. A few months later, more cases were reported in the U.K. Three months before the trial results were published, a Finnish researcher reported that the cause of the outbreak of skin reactions was DMF.[43] What these hundreds of cases had in common was that the people involved had all recently purchased sofas and chairs that were sourced from the same furniture factory in China.[44] The problem was that sachets of DMF had been used as a drying agent to prevent mould. Even as little as one part per million of DMF could cause a severe reaction.[43] Unfortunately, the problem didn't end there. Dermatitis cases were reported in Belgium, France, Ireland, Sweden, Spain and Italy after contact with DMF in furniture, clothing and shoes.[44-47] DMF in leather products such as wallets and handbags also caused significant problems.[48,49]

The concern with DMF causing skin reactions didn't have a direct bearing on the chemical's use in MS, although it would prompt one wag to dub Tecfidera the "poison chair" treatment for MS.[50]

The timing of the sofa scandal may have been unfortunate, but it scarcely slowed plans to develop Tecfidera and two phase III trials were launched. The first was DEFINE (for Determination of the Efficacy and Safety of Oral Fumarate in RRMS), in which 1,234 people with RRMS received one of two doses of DMF or a placebo.[51] The lower doses that had been ineffective in the phase II study were dropped. The dose of 240 mg three times daily was tested again along with a new dose – 240 mg twice daily. Convincing people to take a drug three times a day is a problem so the investigators must have been hoping that twice-daily dosing would be enough. (Once-a-day dosing wasn't feasible because of the drug's very short half-life, which means that after taking a dose, the drug is gone from the body long before the day is over.)

Overall, people in the two Tecfidera groups did much better than expected. During the two years of the study, about 27% had at least one relapse compared to 46% in the placebo group. This corresponded to a 49% lower risk of relapse with treatment. The adjusted ARR was 0.17 with Tecfidera twice-daily, 0.19 with the three times per day dose, and 0.36 with placebo (a reduction of 47-53%). These results surpassed expectations and were a bit surprising. Indeed, even the placebo group in this phase III study outperformed high-dose BG-12 in the phase II study. One reason is undoubtedly the people chosen for the study. DEFINE enrolled people from 28 countries, which can introduce a whole raft of variables, such as accuracy of the diagnosis and access to health care, that may not get factored in. The effect of these differences was seen when different subgroups in the two phase III studies were examined. Eastern Europeans who were enrolled were much less likely to have been treated beforehand for their MS compared to Americans (71% vs. 33%),[52] so one would expect them to have a better response to treatment. And in fact this was the case. In the group of Americans (who represented 15% of participants), Tecfidera reduced the annualized relapse rate by 27-44% – still a substantial amount but considerably less than the 53% reported for the group as a whole.[52]

As in the phase II study, DEFINE appeared to show that Tecfidera had potent effects on the development of new brain lesions seen on MRI. However, these results must be viewed with caution since most people (about 60%) didn't actually have an MRI and we don't know how people were selected for the MRI group. Disability progression, defined as a 1-point increase in the EDSS score that persisted for 12 weeks, was also lower with treatment. Overall, 16-18% of people treated with Tecfidera showed progression compared to 27% in the placebo group. This corresponded to a 34-38% lower risk of progression with Tecfidera at three months (although a more rigorous analysis of 6-month disability progression found no difference with the drug compared to placebo[53]). Curiously enough, the lower dose of Tecfidera was generally more effective than the higher dose – a case of more not being necessarily better.

What are the possible side effects of Tecfidera?

WITH THE 240 MG TWICE-DAILY DOSE (which would later become the approved dose), the most common side effects with Tecfidera were flushing (occurring in 38% of people), diarrhea (15%), nausea (13%) and stomach pain (11%). Adverse effects supposedly diminish over time in many people, but about one in four have persistent problems with flushing.[53] And side effects prompted 16% (about one in six people) to stop taking Tecfidera during the course of the study. Indeed, the number of people who discontinued Tecfidera was very high – about one-third (31%), suggesting that people may have difficulties staying on the drug over the long term.

Serious adverse effects, such as infections or cancers, were rare and no more common with Tecfidera compared to placebo. Fumarates have the potential to be toxic to white blood cells,[54] but low lymphocyte counts were seen in only 4% (but will likely be higher in practice) and didn't appear to be associated with an increased risk of infection. There have been case reports of cancers associated with fumarate use in psoriasis,[55,56] but this link wasn't made in the Tecfidera trial. Fumarates also have the potential to cause kidney damage;[57,58] Tecfidera did have some effects on the kidney but these weren't serious and didn't require stopping the drug. FDA reviewers raised some questions about the possible effects of Tecfidera on the kidney during long-term use,[53] but more studies will be needed to explore this issue.

Periodic urine tests are required during treatment with Tecfidera to ensure that the kidneys are functioning normally.

How does Tecfidera compare with other MS drugs?

A SECOND PHASE III TRIAL of Tecfidera called CONFIRM (for Comparator and an Oral Fumarate in Relapsing–Remitting Multiple Sclerosis) indirectly compared the same two doses of Tecfidera (240 mg twice or three times a day) to Copaxone.[59] Technically speaking, Copaxone was a "reference arm" rather than a direct comparator. What this means essentially is that the researchers wouldn't be obliged to report which treatment was better. The presumed reason was that after the phase II results, the expectation was that Tecfidera and Copaxone would be roughly comparable – reducing relapse rates by about one-third – so it wouldn't be feasible to show that Tecfidera was superior (a very large number of people would be needed to show a difference).[60] Of course the temptation to compare was overwhelming, as we'll see.

Tecfidera was a little less impressive in this second study. Compared to placebo, the risk of having a relapse was reduced 44% with Tecfidera twice-daily (rather than 49% in DEFINE), and 29% with Copaxone (similar to what's been seen in other Copaxone studies). The annualized relapse rate was 0.22 with Tecfidera, 0.29 with Copaxone, and 0.40 with placebo. That meant that ARR was 44% lower with Tecfidera compared to placebo (rather than the 53% seen in DEFINE); and 29% lower with Copaxone versus placebo. The MRI picture also improved with Tecfidera, although the results were somewhat less striking than what was seen in DEFINE. And again, most people didn't have an MRI – a serious shortcoming of the Tecfidera clinical trials program. Neither Tecfidera nor Copaxone significantly reduced the risk of disability progression in this study. This is probably because people in the trial were at an earlier stage of their disease and the rate of disability was low in all groups.

Succumbing to the temptation to compare, the researchers crunched the numbers to see how Tecfidera and Copaxone stacked up. To some, this was something of a straw-man strategy since Copaxone wasn't viewed as an especially potent drug. But as in the REGARD comparison with Rebif, Copaxone was able to hold its own. There were no significant differences between twice-daily Tecfidera and Copaxone with respect to the annualized relapse rate, proportion of people who experienced a relapse on treatment, or time to develop disability. Where Tecfidera differed was on a couple of MRI endpoints. So this was somewhat surprising: in DEFINE, Tecfidera appeared to be as potent as Gilenya or Tysabri, whereas in CONFIRM it was no better than Copaxone.

The same side effects cropped up in CONFIRM that had been seen previously: flushing, diarrhea, nausea and stomach pain. Serious adverse events were uncommon. A recurring theme was the high rate of discontinuations: 30% of people on Tecfidera twice-daily stopped the drug (compared to 25% in the Copaxone group). The most common reason for stopping was side effects such as flushing.

The DEFINE and CONFIRM trial results were the basis for the FDA's approval of Tecfidera in March 2013. The approved indication was for people with relapsing forms of MS[61] (restricted to RRMS in

Canada and other countries[62]). "Relapsing forms" includes not only relapsing-remitting MS but also progressive MS if the person is still experiencing relapses. This is a bit curious since people with progressive MS were specifically excluded from the Tecfidera trials, so the impact of the drug in this group of people isn't known.

Another curiosity is that the FDA safety review didn't address the possible risk of progressive multifocal leukoencephalopathy (PML), which has been such a problem with Tysabri (see Chapter 6). PML is never mentioned, although other health regulators had recommended vigilance[63] because of at least four PML cases that had occurred with either Fumaderm or fumarates.[64]

Unfortunately, one fatal case of PML with Tecfidera was reported in November 2014.[65] The person was in the ENDORSE study (the long-term follow-up of the two phase III studies), and had been taking Tecfidera for four years at the time of death. The reported cause of death was pneumonia. The initial supposition was that the person developed PML because they had long-term suppression of their immune response, which occurs in about 8-10% of people taking Tecfidera.[66] This was also speculated to be the cause of PML in the one case reported with Gilenya. But it is far from clear if this is really the reason. Immunosuppression may be a contributing factor, although a direct cause-and effect relationship between immunosuppression and PML has not been definitively established.[67] Prior immunosuppression contributes to a risk of PML with Tysabri, but doesn't appear to be the actual cause since Tysabri itself doesn't suppress the immune system. So why PML cases have been seen with fumarates needs to be clarified, and this has led to some uncertainties about Tecfidera.

The immediate consequence was a change in the product label, which now includes a warning about the risk of PML.[68] Blood tests are needed every 6-12 months to monitor blood cell counts, and provision has been made to interrupt treatment if white blood cell counts remain persistently low.[68] Regular MRIs may be prudent. In the longer term, it's also likely that doctors will hesitate before switching someone from Tecfidera to Tysabri due to concerns about the PML risk. However, it should be noted that over 100,000 have been exposed to Tecfidera to date, so the PML risk appears to be very low (perhaps 1 in 100,000 rather than 1 in 100 for people with three PML risk factors on Tysabri).

Blood tests have always been a requirement when starting Tecfidera because of the drug's effects on blood cell counts, and periodic tests may be needed to ensure that the drug isn't causing problems with the liver or kidneys. It's best to go off Tecfidera if you're planning to become pregnant (as with all other MS drugs), and to stay off the drug during pregnancy and breastfeeding.

The recommended starting dose is 120 mg twice a day, increased after one week to 240 mg twice a day. This was the regimen used in the clinical trials. We know from the phase II study that the lower dose will not be effective for MS (and may even worsen MS). This sub-effective dose is given to minimize side effects at the start, although there's little evidence that this strategy works.[53]

One problem with taking Tecfidera twice a day is the temptation to take only one capsule, especially if you are experiencing flushing or stomach upset. A half-measure is fine at the beginning, but continuing with this dose – or even taking this dose from time to time – will do little or nothing for your MS. Tecfidera doesn't accumulate in the body, which means that any day you don't take it, there is no MS medication in your system.

The main challenges when starting treatment are flushing and stomach problems. Some people have suggested that taking an Aspirin beforehand will reduce flushing,[69] but the FDA found little evidence for this.[52] Taking the medication with food may reduce the likelihood of vomiting, although this may not have much impact on nausea.[52] Pepto-Bismol doesn't appear to reduce the frequency of stomach upset but may make symptoms somewhat less severe.[70] A U.S. study found that taking Tecfidera with food may help; a majority of people also took some kind of stomach remedy (such as antacids, acid secretion blockers [e.g. Losec], or non-prescription products for nausea, diarrhea, constipation or bloating), which may have provided some relief.[71]

Tecfidera appears to be a solid choice for MS. Its advantages are that it's an oral drug and at least as effective as the injectable medications. Long-term data are unlikely to be helpful. The extension of the DEFINE and CONFIRM studies (called ENDORSE) has reported results after five years on treatment, but these tell us very little since the analysis only included 15% of the original group.[72]

This points to the key disadvantage of Tecfidera. Most people will suffer from side effects, such as flushing and stomach problems, which may or may not get better with time. Tecfidera has the dubious distinction of having the highest drop-out rate seen in clinical trials – and this is an ongoing problem if the depopulated long-term studies are any indication. It has been claimed that the reason for stopping treatment generally isn't side effects such as flushing and stomach upset,[73] but no other explanation has been provided. It remains to be seen how well the drug is tolerated over the long-term course of MS.

CHAPTER 10

WHAT IS AUBAGIO?

A QUARTER-CENTURY AGO, researchers reported that a new chemical called HWA486 (leflunomide) seemed promising as a treatment for autoimmune disorders such as rheumatoid arthritis.[1] Subsequent studies investigated leflunomide for preventing tissue rejection after organ transplantation,[2] and for various autoimmune disorders.[3,4] A decade later, leflunomide (with the brand name Arava) received approval by the FDA for the treatment of rheumatoid arthritis.

Autoimmune disorders and tissue rejection appear dissimilar but they are linked by a common problem. In autoimmune disorders, the immune system mistakes the body's own antigens as foreign and initiates an inflammatory response. A similar thing happens following organ transplantation. The transplanted tissue is identified as foreign (which of course it is) and the body mounts an immune response and "rejects" the new organ. So in autoimmune disease and transplantation, the immune response causes more harm than good and needs to be controlled. What Arava does is inhibit T cells from becoming activated and proliferating,[5,6] in effect stealing some of the spark as the immune system tries to catch fire.

As Arava is broken down in the body it produces a biologically active metabolite called A77 1726. This is the compound that would later be called teriflunomide (brand name Aubagio). Like its parent compound, Aubagio inhibits T cell proliferation.[7] The way it does this is by blocking an enzyme (called dihydro-orotate dehydrogenase) needed to synthesize nucleotides, the building blocks of DNA.[8] In effect, teriflunomide stops immune cells – both T and B cells – from having the raw materials they need to divide. It doesn't have a significant impact on existing immune cells, which can scavenge what they need for ongoing maintenance. So what this means is that as T cells try to proliferate to cause inflammation in the CNS, they can't multiply their numbers. As an aside, at one time it was thought that this drug effect would be useful to treat malaria,[9] but the line of research didn't pan out.

It may also be that Aubagio blocks NF-kappaB (like Tecfidera, see Chapter 9).[10] The effect is to block the switch that turns on the inflammatory signal. So by inhibiting this process, Aubagio has an anti-inflammatory effect.

Aubagio has an unrelated but interesting effect on bone. Bone is constantly being recycled by the body, with some cells breaking down bone and others acting to rebuild it; osteoporosis occurs when this balance is lost. Aubagio appears to inhibit the breakdown of bone,[11] which may be one of the reasons why its parent compound, Arava, may prevent joint destruction in rheumatoid arthritis. This side benefit may make it attractive to people with MS with early osteoporosis.

Yet another effect was discovered a decade ago, which created some interest in developing Aubagio as an MS therapy. Astrocytes are a type of cell found in the brain and spinal cord; when stimulated, they produce an inflammatory chemical (nitric oxide, one of the free radicals discussed in Chapter 9) that harms brain tissue. Laboratory studies suggested that Arava could inhibit this inflammatory process in the brain,[12] which in turn hinted at a role in MS.

This line of research was never pursued for Arava, perhaps because pricing for Arava had already been established and it would be more lucrative to start from scratch with a new drug (European regulators initially ruled that Aubagio wasn't a "new active substance" but only a breakdown product of leflunomide, a decision that was later reversed[13]). So Aubagio was the drug selected for the phase II study in RRMS or relapsing secondary-progressive MS.[14] Most people were recruited from Canada. The bioavailability (the amount of drug that is usable by the body) of leflunomide is 70%, which means that doses of 10 mg and 20 mg of leflunomide are the same as 7 mg and 14 mg of Aubagio.[15] While the dosing used for rheumatoid arthritis isn't necessarily ideal for MS, these were the Aubagio doses used in the phase II study. The researchers found that Aubagio reduced MS activity seen on MRI by about 60% during the 36-week study, but it did not significantly affect the relapse rate. A long-term follow-up of the study suggested that Aubagio kept working over 5-6 years,[16] although any firm conclusions are difficult to make since many people stopped the trial early.

How effective is Aubagio in MS?

THESE RESULTS LED TO TWO PHASE III STUDIES called TEMSO and TOWER. In TEMSO (for Teriflunomide MS Oral), over one thousand people with MS received Aubagio 7 mg or 14 mg per day or placebo for two years.[17] Both doses of Aubagio were effective in reducing inflammatory activity on MRI, as the phase II study had already shown. With the larger number of people in TEMSO, Aubagio was able to show that it reduced the relapse rate by 31-32%; this is about what is seen with Betaseron or Rebif (with the usual caveat about comparing one trial with another). There was some effect on disability with high-dose Aubagio but not with the lower dose. People outside of North America did somewhat better than North Americans;[18] this was also seen in a Tecfidera trial, and can probably be attributed to the people selected for the study. In the ongoing extension of TEMSO, relapse rates have remained low after up to nine years of treatment.[19]

TOWER (for Teriflunomide Oral in people with Relapsing MS) was the second phase III study used to get FDA approval and was very similar to TEMSO. Over one thousand people received 7 mg or 14 mg of Aubagio or a placebo. An unusual feature was that MRIs were not obtained. The higher dose of Aubagio lowered the relapse rate by about 36% (so somewhat better than what is seen with interferons) and reduced disability progression by about 32%.[20] However, the 7-mg dose was unimpressive: the relapse rate was reduced only 22% and there was no effect on disability. Despite this, the FDA approved the 7-mg dose in 2012; the lower dose was not approved in Canada.

Thus, the 14-mg dose of Aubagio appears to be effective; the 7 mg dose doesn't provide much benefit. The impression that the effect of Aubagio is comparable to what has been seen with the injectables was confirmed in two additional studies. In the TOPIC trial of CIS,[21] the two doses of Aubagio lowered the risk of developing MS by 37-43% – very similar to the results of the CIS studies of the interferons and Copaxone.

Aubagio was directly compared to Rebif in the phase III TENERE trial.[22] The main endpoint of the study was downright odd: treatment failure, defined as a relapse or discontinuation of the drug. With respect to treatment failure, neither of the medications did very well. Just over 40% of people met the criteria for treatment failure while on either Aubagio 14 mg or Rebif. Indeed, about 25% failed in the first six months with either treatment. In terms of relapse rates, people taking either dose of Aubagio were more likely to have a relapse than if they were on Rebif. However, people generally preferred to take Aubagio because it was more convenient and side effects were more tolerable.

Aubagio does appear to be very well tolerated. The most common side effects are infections (such as the flu or urinary tract infections), gastrointestinal disorders (such as diarrhea and nausea), and hair thinning. A pooled safety analysis of all three phase III studies found nothing new or alarming.[23] There can be small increases in blood pressure so it's important to take your blood pressure from time to time.

The FDA flagged a potential for liver effects with Aubagio. This hasn't been a common problem with Aubagio but has occurred with its parent compound. So blood tests are needed periodically to ensure that the drug doesn't cause liver damage. A second issue is numbness or tingling, which occurred in about 10-11% of people taking Aubagio. Since this is a common symptom of MS, it's difficult to determine if this is a drug-related side effect or is MS-related or, alternatively, if MS is masking the frequency of this effect.

Aubagio has a potential to affect a developing fetus, although this risk appears to be low; a follow-up of 30 babies exposed to the drug found no abnormalities and birth weights were normal.[24] But to be on the safe side, if a woman becomes pregnant while on the drug, a special procedure (a regimen of either cholestyramine or activated charcoal) is needed to remove the drug from the body as quickly as possible. Otherwise it will take several months to clear the body (or years in some cases), which is too long a time for a fetus to be exposed to the drug. Cholestyramine is granules that can be mixed with fruit juice or sprinkled over cereal, so it isn't especially unpleasant to take. It isn't absorbed by the body, but is a resin that binds to substances in the body to eliminate them. The 11-day course removes virtually all of the Aubagio from the body, which may provide some reassurance to someone who is planning to become pregnant. An unusual situation is that men taking Aubagio are also advised to undergo this special drug-removal procedure if they are planning to father a child since the drug is detectable in semen (it's the only MS drug found in semen).

So Aubagio provides another treatment option – especially for people about to start therapy who aren't keen on injections. Approvals were quickly obtained from the "A" list – America, Australia and

Argentina. Canada granted approval in late 2013, so no doubt the drug will quickly work its way through the alphabet of countries.

The chief advantages of Aubagio are that it's an oral drug and it seems to be easily tolerated, so it's likely to become one of the preferred medications for starting treatment. A few preliminary studies have suggested that exposure to Aubagio and an injectable doesn't cause any harm,[25,26] so people who are tired of injections and want something simpler to take can probably switch directly to Aubagio. A phase III study called TERACLES[27] planned to examine the combination of Aubagio with an injectable but the trial was cancelled, no doubt because it's unlikely that someone would take both an oral and an injectable therapy at the same time.

CHAPTER 11

WHAT IS LEMTRADA?

ALEMTUZUMAB (branded as lemtrada in MS) is the most recent treatment approved for MS but one that was in development for three decades before finding a home.

In the 1970s, a technique was described to grow large numbers of cells of a specific type that would produce antibodies capable of binding to key targets (antigens).[1,2] In effect, a cell's machinery was recruited to manufacture a specific biological product. The targeted nature of these monoclonal antibodies (MAbs) meant that doctors could take aim at a given protein involved in a disease process. The first MAb drug approved for MS was Tysabri, in which the target is an adhesion molecule (alpha4-integrin) that allows activated immune cells (T cells) to stick to the wall of blood vessels prior to crossing over into the central nervous system.

Lemtrada uses the same technology as Tysabri but has a different target. It was developed in the 1980s in the U.K. and its name – Campath-1 – was derived from its birthplace, the Cambridge Pathology lab.[3] First tested in a woman with a form of anemia, it was later discovered that Campath-1H (the H meant it had been "humanized", i.e. derived in part from human as well as non-human sources) was targeting a specific protein (called CD52) on the surface of immune cells (including T cells), which appeared to cause the cells to self-destruct,[4] although the purpose and function of CD52 is still poorly understood. (The drug was later found to target B cells as well.) Destroying lymphocytes (white blood cells, including T and B cells) was very useful in fighting certain types of leukemia (in which there are too many white blood cells). So the British National Research and Development Council (later renamed the British Technology Group) acquired the rights to commercialize Campath.

Thus would begin a long process of "hot-potato" development.[3,5] Campath-1H was licensed to Wellcome Biotech, which became Wellcome, which then merged with Glaxo to form Glaxo-Wellcome. Glaxo-Wellcome planned to bring Campath-1H to market as a leukemia treatment but crunched a few numbers, didn't like the sound they made, and pulled the plug on the program in 1994. A start-up biotech company, Leukosite, acquired Campath, then partnered with another biotech, ILEX, to develop the drug. They joined forces with Schering and succeeded in obtaining FDA approval for Campath in 2001 as a treatment for a type of leukemia.

But this was far from the end of the story. Leukosite was bought out by Millennium Pharmaceuticals, which sold its share of Campath-1H to ILEX. Campath-1H then went from one Cambridge to another when ILEX was bought by Genzyme, an American biotech based in

Cambridge, Massachusetts. In 2011, Genzyme was acquired by Sanofi-Aventis (later just Sanofi), itself an agglomeration of a half-dozen drug companies.

Throughout this process, Campath-1H was being investigated as a possible treatment for autoimmune disorders. In 1991, a neurologist in Cambridge (England) tried using it in a woman who was confined to a wheelchair because of her MS. Within a few months she was reportedly able to go skiing.[5] An MRI showed that the inflammation in her brain was substantially reduced. This salutary report prompted a small pilot study of Campath-1H in 14 people with MS in 1996.[6] MS activity on MRI was greatly reduced, although most found that their MS symptoms initially got worse,[7] an effect that could be offset somewhat by an initial course of steroids. Another concern was that Campath-1H had a potent effect on T cells, and about one-third of people developed a new autoimmune disorder, which most often affected the thyroid.[8]

So Campath-1H was a very potent drug. A single dose could reduce inflammatory activity on MRI by up to 90%.[9] Five days of treatment reduced the body's circulating T cells by 95%, and the T cell population didn't recover for over 18 months.[10] (A later study indicated that it may take three years for T cells to recover[11]) However, despite its powerful effect on inflammation, about one-half of people continued to have worsening disability,[9] and the drug provided little or no benefit in progressive MS.[12]

The potency of Campath-1 suggested it might have a role in people with highly active MS[13] – frequent, severe relapses that don't respond well enough to the usual injection drugs. At the time there were few good options. One possibility was mitoxantrone (Novantrone), approved in some countries for use in MS, but this could only be used for a short time because cumulative doses were toxic to the heart.

The potential benefits – and the potential risks – of Campath-1 were seen in the CAMMS223 (for Campath-1H in MS) trial.[14] In this phase II trial, 334 people with early MS received either one of two doses of Campath-1H or Rebif (there was no placebo group). The study was a bit different in a couple of respects. It was scheduled to last three years (phase II studies are often only a year). And the dosing of Campath-1H was infrequent: five days of the drug given by infusion (a slow drip into the vein) in the first year, followed by three more days of treatment in each of the subsequent years (so a total of 11 days of treatment over three years). As it turned out, after most people had received the second course of treatment, the trial was stopped because of safety concerns. The reason was that three people developed ITP (for immune thrombocytopenic purpura), an autoimmune condition in which blood platelets are destroyed and the person develops bruising and bleeding complications. One person died. Three additional cases of ITP were later discovered.

Despite this unfortunate turn of events, the researchers were impressed with their data. Campath-1H reduced the relapse rate by 74% compared to Rebif; the average relapse rate was 0.10 with Campath-1H versus 0.36 with Rebif. Overall, 80% of people taking Campath-1H experienced no relapses over the three-year period compared to 52% of those on Rebif. MRI results were less than expected, although Campath-1H was better than Rebif on this measure as well.

Perhaps most surprising was the effect of the drug on disability outcomes. The risk of disability progression was reduced by two-thirds with Campath-1H compared to Rebif. In real numbers, this meant that people improved slightly on their EDSS score with Campath-1H (from an average EDSS score of 2.0 to about 1.6), and worsened slightly while on Rebif (from 1.9 to about 2.3). Indeed, previous studies hadn't given any indication that Campath-1H would have much effect on disability. This impact on disability was attributed, as one might expect, to a possible neuroprotective effect of the drug.[15]

Neuroprotective or not, safety was an issue. In addition to the death from ITP, three people were diagnosed with cancer (compared to 1 in the Rebif group), a possible "safety signal" that needed to be watched. About one in four developed thyroid problems. Almost everyone had some kind of reaction to the infusion (most commonly rash, headache, fever and fatigue). And two-thirds developed an infection, such as a respiratory infection, urinary tract infection, herpes (cold sores) or vaginitis.

Results at the five-year mark were remarkably similar. The average relapse rate remained low (0.11) and the risk of disability progression was about 72% lower with Campath-1H compared to Rebif.[16] This indicated that Campath-1H was still having an effect even though people hadn't taken the drug for two or three years. But it also meant that there was an ongoing need to monitor safety even years after the last dose of Campath-1H (and years after the drug had been eliminated from the person's body) because there was still a risk of developing side effects.

Fortunately there were no cases of progressive multifocal leukoencephalopathy (PML) in the study. PML has been reported in people treated with Campath-1H for other conditions (not MS).[17,18] A Canadian survey of PML in people receiving a MAb found that about 8% of cases were in people receiving Campath-1H (compared to 18% of cases for Tysabri).[19] So the risk is not negligible, but the factors that contribute to this risk in people with MS haven't been determined yet. As of February 2015, no PML cases have been reported in people with MS treated with the drug.

The CAMMS223 trial was the swansong for Campath-1H. Its MAb moniker, alemtuzumab (soon to be branded as Lemtrada), became the preferred term as development continued in MS. The next step was to launch two large-scale trials under the banner of a Comparison of Alemtuzumab and Rebif Efficacy in Multiple Sclerosis (CARE-MS).

How effective is Lemtrada in MS?

WHILE THIS WAS UNDERWAY and before any phase III results were known to the general public, Sanofi made a surprising move and pulled Campath-1H off the market. This was highly controversial since the drug was an effective treatment for people with leukemia. But the thinking was that the lower-priced Campath needed to make way for the planned launch of Lemtrada. As an MS drug, Lemtrada could be priced in line with as other newly-minted MS drugs, and withdrawing

Campath-1H would keep it out of the hands of people tempted to use Campath-1H off-label for MS.[20] [It's important to note that Campath is used at a much higher dose for cancer than Lemtrada is for MS.] To quiet concerns about the fate of leukemia patients, Sanofi agreed to make Campath-1H available free of charge to the people who needed it.

These manoeuverings worked off the assumption that Lemtrada would be successful in the phase III studies. These results were published a few months later in November 2012. Both of the CARE-MS studies compared Lemtrada with Rebif. The difference between the two studies was the people enrolled: CARE-MS I studied those newly-diagnosed with MS,[21] whereas CARE-MS II included people who had been previously treated with another MS drug (mostly an interferon or Copaxone, although a few had previously been on Tysabri).[22] The dosing schedule of Lemtrada was the same as in the phase II study: five days of infusions, then another three infusions a year later. Everyone also received a short course of steroids to guard against symptoms getting worse at the time of the infusion.[7] About a year into the study, an antiviral drug was added in an effort to prevent an emerging problem of herpes flare-ups during treatment.

When designing the studies, an unusual decision was not to include a placebo group. Efforts were made to "double-blind" the study, i.e. the investigators and the people in the study didn't know which treatment was being administered (which can bias the results). But this wasn't really possible with these medications since they produce very distinctive side effects.

A further problem was that the results of the phase II study were announced just as people were starting the phase III program – creating more room for bias since the people in the trial the drug could read about the new drug in the newspaper.[24] Complaints about how these studies were conducted would crop up later in the FDA's initial review of the drug development program.

People in the CARE-MS I trial had been living with MS for fewer than five years but had active disease – an average of two relapses a year and mild disability (EDSS 2.0) at the outset. With the more rigorous conditions of the phase III trial, Lemtrada was not quite as effective as it was in the phase II study – but the results were certainly impressive enough. The average relapse rate fell to 0.18 compared to 0.39 with Rebif, meaning it was about 55% better than an active MS drug (i.e. not a placebo). Overall, 78% of people taking Lemtrada had no relapses compared to 59% with Rebif (a relative difference of 32%). Lemtrada also bested Rebif with respect to inflammatory activity on MRI, although not quite as robustly as in previous studies. A surprising finding was that Lemtrada was no better than Rebif on disability progression: 8% showed some progression with Lemtrada compared to 11% with Rebif. This is likely explained by the very low rates of progression seen in this cohort of people. Both drug groups showed a very small improvement in their EDSS scores.

People in the Lemtrada group experienced more side effects than those taking Rebif, although few people stopped treatment because of them. (Of course, "stopping therapy" is a little tricky to define when a drug is taken for only a few days a year.) The most common side effects with Lemtrada were headache, rash, fever, nausea, fatigue, skin reactions and flushing. Almost everyone experienced some kind of reaction during the Lemtrada infusion, although only 3% of these were serious. Infections were quite common but most were mild to moderate in severity. About one in six people developed a herpes infection (e.g. cold sores or genital herpes) despite the use of antiviral drugs by many in the study.

A minority of people experienced severe side effects. One person died after developing an autoimmune blood disorder over a year after taking the last dose of Lemtrada. Only 1% developed ITP. Thyroid disease occurred in about one in five people on Lemtrada.

CARE-MS I was the first hurdle Lemtrada had to overcome but the study wasn't really reflective of real life: few people with early MS would receive such a potent drug within the first few years of being diagnosed. But there was a second study, CARE-MS II, to examine what happens in people in whom a previous MS drug had failed.[22] Two doses of Lemtrada (12 and 24 milligrams) were tested, although the higher dose was later dropped when it became too difficult to recruit people into the study. A criterion for being included was that everyone had to have experienced at least one relapse while on another drug. Since a single relapse on a therapy doesn't necessarily mean that a treatment is ineffective, it's fair to say that about one-half of the study participants hadn't really experienced a "treatment failure", although they did appear to have fairly active disease. Most people had been taking an interferon, one-third had been on Copaxone and a few had taken Tysabri. About one in four had tried more than one drug. On average, people had been on therapy for about three years when the study started. As in the other CARE-MS study, people also received a course of steroids as well as an antiviral drug.

The people in CARE-MS II had more intractable MS so perhaps it isn't surprising that they didn't do quite as well as those in CARE-MS I. In fact, one-third of people taking Lemtrada continued having relapses. Overall, the average number of relapses per year was 0.26 with Lemtrada compared to 0.52 with Rebif, meaning the relative risk of relapse was 50% lower with Lemtrada. One factor to consider, however, was that most people in the Rebif group had already been on an interferon and hadn't done especially well, so the comparison isn't entirely fair. There was no difference between the two treatments in the volume of lesions seen on MRI, but Lemtrada was more effective in shutting down new lesion formation in the brain.

An important finding was that CARE-MS II was able to show that Lemtrada had a greater effect on disability progression – 42% lower with Lemtrada compared to Rebif. In real terms, people taking Lemtrada showed a small improvement in their EDSS (an average of 0.17 points), whereas those taking Rebif showed a slight worsening (on average about 0.24 points). While it would be tempting to extrapolate from the results that a 0.17 improvement might result in a 1-point difference in EDSS score in as little as six years (0.17 x 6=1.02), this is probably too much to expect. In the two-year extension of CARE-MS II (during which a majority of people were not re-dosed), disability was stable or improved in about two-thirds of people.[23] This included a group (about 15%) who were somewhat better than they'd been at the start of the study. So these were remarkably good results, especially considering that the medication seemed to have a sustained benefit even two years after people stopped taking it.

Safety issues were similar to what was seen in the other phase III trial. Ninety percent experienced a side effect when the drug was infused; the most common were headache, rash, other skin reactions, nausea or fever. Three-quarters of people taking Lemtrada developed some kind of infection, most often respiratory-related or urinary tract infections. About 16% developed a thyroid disorder from the drug. And again, one in six had a herpes infection, such as cold sores, genital herpes or shingles – despite the fact that most were taking an antiviral medication at the time. It isn't clear what proportion of these were new herpes infections. It's pretty safe to assume that most (and certainly all of the shingles cases) were due to reactivation of the virus, a result of treatment suppressing the immune system that normally keeps the virus in check. About 4% had a serious infection (such as pneumonia), and 1% developed ITP.

There were three cancers in the Lemtrada group (including one thyroid cancer), and two cancers in the Rebif group. These numbers are low, but a possible cancer risk was flagged by the FDA in its November 2013 review.[24] That report noted that while the incidence of thyroid cancer was very low (0.4%), the rate was higher than what is seen in the general population. The incidence of melanoma was also three-fold higher in people treated with Lemtrada, although absolute numbers were low.[24] But it suggested that it might be prudent to have your moles checked by a dermatologist every so often (and generally advised for anyone because of the rising rates of melanoma).

The FDA also noted that 2.5% of people experienced serious infusion reactions, and there is a risk of infections while on the drug.[24] Another concern was the ITP already mentioned, which can cause fatal bleeding complications. The incidence of ITP (about 4.4 cases per 1000 patient-years) in clinical trials of Lemtrada was low, but higher than what is seen in the general population.[24]

Why did the FDA delay approval of Lemtrada?

THE SAFETY CONCERNS raised by the FDA were only part of the story. The other part of the risk-benefit equation is benefit, and here there were additional problems. The FDA had wanted the phase III studies to include a placebo group as a comparison, but this wasn't done. And the way the studies were set up created biases and raised questions in the collective mind of the FDA. "The issues arisen from the two studies are beyond the scope of statistics," one reviewer stated. "The only way to solve the issues raised in this review is to conduct fresh new studies."[24]

The risks were fairly well known; the benefits were uncertain, at least to the FDA staff. As a result, the three FDA reviewers voted against the approval of Lemtrada. One person did not recommend approval because of safety issues unless substantial benefits could be shown, and two said that there wasn't enough good evidence to show that the drug was effective.[24]

This nay-saying wasn't seen in other countries. In the latter half of 2013, the drug did receive approval in Europe, Australia and

Canada. To the European Medicines Agency, the benefits clearly outweighed any risks associated with the drug.[25]

These approvals fuelled some dissention in the ranks of the FDA. The FDA's Peripheral and Central Nervous System Drugs Advisory Committee found the EMA's appraisal more compelling than the FDA's own report, and recommended approval of the drug. But when it came time to pick the winning horse, the vote came up camels. The FDA stated that the trials weren't good enough to enable them to evaluate the drug, but agreed that there was substantial evidence of the drug's benefits.[26] So they didn't like the trials, did like the trial data, but not quite enough. The unanimous conclusion was that the risks of Lemtrada should not prevent its approval in the U.S. for the treatment of relapsing MS.[26]

But at the eleventh hour, on the day before New Year's Eve, the FDA did exactly that. It sided with its own staff rather than its expert committee, and ruled that Lemtrada could not be marketed in the U.S.

The manufacturer decided not to appeal the FDA decision, but it also announced that it had no intention of doing new studies – which would take years to complete and cost millions of dollars. Instead, they re-submitted the same studies in May 2014 but with new analyses and some long-term data to bolster their case.

Perhaps those data were especially compelling. Or perhaps the FDA listened to the outcry from patient groups and physicians about the need to have a big gun in the MS arsenal. For the FDA reversed its decision in December 2014, allowing Lemtrada to be used as an MS treatment in the U.S., with the caveat that close monitoring was required to address potential safety concerns. People needed to be watched for two hours at the time of their infusion. Monthly blood tests were needed for 48 months after the last dose, a urine sample was required every three months, and skin exams were needed annually (although the risk of skin cancer is estimated to be less than 1%).

The FDA-approval label also stated that Lemtrada should generally be reserved for people who had not responded well enough to two prior MS therapies. This contrasts with the drug label in other countries. In Canada, Lemtrada can be used earlier – after only one prior therapy has been shown to be ineffective. In Europe, Lemtrada can be used as the initial MS therapy. This is called an induction strategy, a term borrowed from cancer chemotherapy. It means using a heavy-hammer treatment to produce a rapid, profound response, which can then be maintained by a less powerful drug. Tysabri was once touted as a possible induction therapy, although it really isn't suited for this purpose because of the difficulties in stopping the drug. Arguably, Lemtrada isn't a true induction agent either. Induction is meant to be a short-term strategy, and a few doses of Lemtrada will produce effects on the immune system for years to come. But some may decide to try one or two courses of Lemtrada as a means of "re-setting" the abnormal immune response – in effect, rebooting the immune system – then start another drug later on to maintain that response. But it's important to note that this approach hasn't been studied yet. It isn't known if it will be safe to go from Lemtrada to another drug, nor if another drug can maintain the effectiveness.

For some, Lemtrada is seen as a much-valued treatment of last resort. For those people who have continued to worsen on other MS therapies, there's a chance that they'll respond to Lemtrada. It provides a flicker of hope. That is probably reason enough to justify a place for Lemtrada on the list of treatment options. However, an emerging idea is to use Lemtrada earlier in the course of treatment. For if we accept the notion that early treatment is better, then a potent readjustment of the abnormal immune response up front may have the greatest impact on the long-term course of MS. If MS is a long path heading to a future of disability, a quick push off the path when you first set out may be more likely to take you somewhere different. Such an argument is theoretical at the moment (although it has been used to justify stem-cell transplants in MS). It remains to be seen if early induction with Lemtrada can reduce the risk of disability later on.

THESE NEWER TREATMENTS – oral Aubagio and the infusion drug Lemtrada – have yet to define their place in the treatment scheme. They will jostle for position with the oral drugs Gilenya and Tecfidera, and the infusion drug Tysabri, as part of the next-generation MS therapies. With four injection drugs, three oral drugs and two infusion drugs available now (with more therapies to come), there is a wealth of treatment options for MS.

In the final chapter we'll look at some of the things to consider when choosing the best therapy for your MS.

CHAPTER 12

HOW DO I CHOOSE A THERAPY?

OVER THE COURSE OF TWO DECADES, the MS community has gone from having no treatments to having nine: Avonex, Betaseron/Extavia, Rebif, Copaxone, Tysabri, Gilenya, Aubagio, Lemtrada and Novantrone. Many claims have been made for all of these medications, but it's important to appreciate why you're starting a treatment in the first place, what a therapy can do and, just as importantly, what a medication can't do for your MS. In this chapter we'll summarize how the drugs compare with one another, and how the wealth of treatment choices can best be used to expand your options in the years ahead.

Why treat MS?

THE REASONING behind all of the MS medications is based on three simple premises: that the inflammation and damage that occurs is primarily due to a disordered immune response; modulating this response with a drug that targets inflammation will produce short-term benefits; and that this reduction in inflammatory damage will result in less disability over the longer term.

The first-generation injectables do reduce the frequency of relapses and the amount of inflammation in the brain and spinal cord. However, it is my no means certain whether these drugs can slow the development of disability over the long-term and, if they do, whether their impact is enough. So it's certainly fair to question whether their modest benefits are worth all the time and trouble of injecting yourself on a regular basis.

It's equally fair to ask if the new-generation medications will prove to be any more effective in controlling the disease process and slowing the progression of disability. All of these treatments – the oral medications (Aubagio, Tecfidera and Gilenya) and the infusion agents (Tysabri, Lemtrada) – use the same approach of targeting inflammation, and work off the assumption that more is better. More anti-inflammatory action will mean more benefit down the road. Certainly the newer medications are generally more potent in modulating the immune system than the injectables. What remains to be established is if this short-term benefit (fewer relapses, less activity on MRI) will translate into fewer or less severe impairments during long-term treatment. Indeed, it still needs to be determined if any medication that primarily influences immune dysregulation in this way will have a significant impact on the neurodegenerative processes that cause a permanent loss of neurological function. This is the most important question in MS research today.

MUCH ATTENTION HAS BEEN PAID to the relative benefits and risks of treatment – and it's essential that everyone weigh these before choosing a treatment. But before we address this issue in more detail, we should pause to consider the known risks associated with MS itself.

The MS disease process is a slow burn. Relapses are the most obvious sign that there's inflammation in the CNS, but these are just periodic flare-ups of a smouldering inflammation that is causing ongoing damage to the delicate tissues of the brain and spinal cord. The body is able to repair some of the damage during periods of remission, but it's a losing battle. You cannot renovate if the house is still on fire.

As we saw earlier, natural history studies have shown that left untreated, relapsing-remitting MS will develop into secondary-progressive MS in about 85% of cases. Over time, relapses will slowly diminish in severity and frequency, which can give the false impression that MS has gone into remission. Unfortunately, the disease continues to cause damage. Over the course of twenty years or so, the losses in function that were once temporary will likely become permanent, and they will start to accumulate. That means that the various symptoms that can strike you – muscle weakness, numbness, bowel/bladder symptoms – will become part of your daily life. These impairments will become "the new normal".

When you're first diagnosed, it's certainly tempting to push the diagnosis to the back of your mind into the realm of unreality, especially if your symptoms go away and you feel more or less normal again. Some problems go away without the need to do anything. But this isn't the case with MS. Time won't heal the wounds.

The best time to start treatment is soon after you've been diagnosed. This is when inflammation is at its worst, and when treatments – which target this inflammation – are probably most effective. Inflammation is the match that ignites the burn, but that match becomes less and less important once the fire has been kindled. After that, the damage to CNS tissues – the nerve fibres, the myelin that protects them and the cells that maintain them – is probably a self-sustaining process that is largely independent of inflammation. The initial immune dysfunction probably starts a cascade of other immune reactions in the CNS so that neurodegeneration will continue even if there are no more inflammatory flare-ups. This is what's seen in primary-progressive MS, in which disability begins to accumulate from the outset even though relapses are infrequent or absent. It's also seen in people with relapsing-remitting MS once they've reached the secondary-progressive phase, and most people will reach that phase.

If you're diagnosed with relapsing-remitting MS rather than progressive MS, you may have a bit more time to decide on your best course of action. But don't be lulled into a false sense of security. The divide between relapsing-remitting and progressive forms of MS is an artificial one. Relapsing-remitting MS *is* progressive MS, or will be. The symptoms may remit, but the disease will not. That is why it needs to be treated. And the best hope for treatment is to start before the disease process gains momentum – when there's still the possibility that it can be deflected from its course of irreversible disability.

How do I choose the best treatment?

SELECTING THE RIGHT TREATMENT will be an ongoing process because there's no one drug that's best for everyone. It may require some trial and error. But a good plan today is better than a perfect plan tomorrow.

There are two general approaches to starting a treatment. The first is to start slowly, using a medication that is somewhat effective, and keeping the big guns in reserve. This is how doctors typically use antibiotics. If you have a sinus infection or bronchitis, they'll prescribe a penicillin-type drug (e.g. a cephalosporin) knowing that these medications will clear the infection in most cases. If the bug is resistant or you can't tolerate the drug, they'll switch to a more effective treatment. Of course MS isn't an acute illness like bronchitis, and the disease doesn't become resistant to treatment, so the medical paradigm (the models that doctors use as a way of thinking about disease) doesn't entirely suit the circumstances. But this approach made sense when the injectables were the only option, and we'll continue to see this strategy as Aubagio and Tecfidera become more widely available.

The second approach is more in keeping with the chemotherapy paradigm. This model sees illness as a threat that cannot go unchecked, so the approach is to treat it early and hit it hard with the most effective drug to knock the illness into remission. You don't use a moderately effective drug to treat cancer – you use the best weapons in the arsenal. The risk, of course, is that the treatment can cause problems of its own, but this can be justified for a fatal illness like cancer. The question is if this aggressive approach can be justified for a chronic rather than fatal illness, such as MS.

How you view these strategies – the "antibiotic approach" versus the "chemotherapy approach" – will be influenced by how you view your MS. Do you see your MS as if it were diabetes: a chronic illness that requires daily care and which has a risk of long-term impairments? Or do you think of it as a serious threat to your day-to-day life and how you imagined your future, so it needs to be met with fierce resistance?

There isn't a correct answer to these questions, and how you view things will be influenced in part by how severe your illness is at the moment. Perhaps many people will find themselves somewhere between these two extremes, while others will shift their position over time. The goal here is not to dictate how you should feel about MS, but rather to provide a framework so you and your doctor can decide what treatment is best for you.

A reasonable strategy when considering treatment is to think of a five-year plan. The plan should try to address four key questions:

- Which is the best drug for my circumstances (i.e. my present level of disease severity and my risk of future disability)?
- Can I live with the side effects (because all treatments have side effects) or will they stop me from staying on the medication?
- Is my treatment working?
- What will be the second-choice drug? Many people won't fully respond to the first-choice drug so a second drug will often be

needed. It's important that the first drug in the sequence doesn't limit your options for a second drug.

What is the best drug for my circumstances?

WE WOULD ALL LIKE TO PERSONALIZE our choice of medication, using the one that's best suited to our circumstances. MS would seem to be a good candidate for individualized medicine: it strikes people at different times in their lives, creates a cluster of symptoms that are unique to the individual, and it has differing clinical courses. In an ideal world there would be tests to show who is at risk of developing early disability, who will have a more benign course, who will respond to a specific therapy, and who isn't responding well enough to a medication. These tests don't exist. So neurologists have to make some inferences based on the specifics of your MS.

When you are first diagnosed, your prognosis will be largely based on the factors that indicate that your MS is more active and/or you have a higher risk of progression. This is how family doctors view your risk of a heart attack: they'll measure blood pressure and lipid levels, test for diabetes, ask about smoking, and so on. In other words, they'll do a risk assessment. But bear in mind that these are risks, not inevitabilities.

There are six main factors at the beginning that suggest a higher risk of more active or progressive MS. Three of these relate to you as a person and can't be modified: your sex, age and ethnicity. There's a higher risk if you are male, older when first diagnosed, and of African ancestry.

Three of the factors relate to the specifics of your MS: the severity of your relapses; how inflammatory your disease process is; and how well you recover from relapses. Frequent relapses, severe relapses, and poor recovery from a relapse – intuitively these seem like bad signs, and in fact they are predictive of greater disability in the future.[1-4] Severe relapses suggest a more dysregulated immune response and a more aggressive inflammatory process that needs to be brought under control. The lesions seen on MRI demonstrate in a very visual way that there is ongoing inflammation in the brain, so it's a warning sign of disease activity.[5] But note that over time, relapses aren't a good long-term indicator of your risk of developing secondary-progressive MS.[6] As you go along, relapses become less useful in predicting what the long-term course will be.

Relapse recovery is about the body's ability to re-regulate the immune response, cool down the inflammation and heal the damage. There are doubtless many factors involved, but how these factors come into play and interact with other factors is largely unknown. It's unclear why the immune response is dysregulated in the first place, so it is far from clear how to bring it back to normal. Part of the problem is undoubtedly inflammation, which creates a toxic microenvironment in the brain that impedes remyelination of damaged myelin and causes damage to the cells needed for nerve function. Targeting some of the known players involved in the inflammatory response may help fine-tune this approach in the future. Attention is currently focused on ways to stop particularly aggressive T cells (such as Th17), stimulate T cells that are known to regulate the immune response (called Tregs), and promote factors involved in remyelination and repair.

Following a relapse, the brain and spinal cord are vulnerable to a new immune attack. This is one reason why frequent relapses are important to your risk of progression. During the period in between relapses (the time of remission), the body tries to fix the damage. A new inflammatory flare-up is the dirt in the wound that makes it more difficult for your body to repair itself. Healing is generally better in younger people, which may be one reason why people tend to progress more quickly if they are diagnosed when they are older. Genetic factors also influence a person's ability to heal, but what these factors are is largely a mystery at the moment.

So frequent, severe relapses, ongoing inflammation (as evidenced by persistent symptoms and new lesions on your MRI), and poor recovery from relapses are early warning signs. Ongoing inflammation (relapses and MRI activity) is especially important once you start a treatment. In part, this is because it shows that the problem is persisting despite treatment, but also because it indicates that the medication isn't working effectively enough. At the very least, MS medications must control inflammation – that is their main purpose – and if there is still ongoing inflammation in the brain (relapses, new MRI lesions), the treatment isn't doing its job.

These risk factors are important to consider when thinking about starting an MS treatment. Individual risk factors haven't been weighted, so it isn't known which are the more important. Nor is it known how these risks interact, although it's probably fair to assume that more risk factors translate to a worse situation down the road.

As a general rule, people with milder disease at the beginning often choose a less potent medication, such as one of the injectables (interferons or Copaxone), Aubagio or Tecfidera. For more aggressive disease, it may be better to start with Gilenya, Tysabri or Lemtrada. This assumes that all treatment options are available in your country and your insurer will reimburse them. If Gilenya, Tysabri or Lemtrada isn't available to you right away (either because of regulations in your country or your insurer doesn't cover it), you'll need to start with one of the other therapies.

As the drug studies summarized in the previous chapters should show, no MS drug works in everyone and no MS therapy is the "best" choice.[7] Your MS is as unique as you are, so you and your neurologist need to work together to determine what's best according to your circumstances. The decision about which medication to start will be based on your weighing of the pros and cons, the benefits and risks, with the options available to you. The severity of your illness is part of the equation, but you'll also need to consider what's important to you, your values and lifestyle. It's your life and your body, so ultimately the decision of which treatment to take – and to keep taking – will rest with you.

How do the first-choice medications compare?

THE PREVIOUS CHAPTERS provide the specifics of how the different MS medications fared in clinical trials. It would be nice to know how they stack up against one another, but there have been few head-to-head studies directly comparing the different medications.

A few studies have shown that Betaseron, Rebif and Copaxone have a very similar impact on relapses.[8-10] So the choice of one injectable over another will largely be determined by your preferences with respect to the frequency of injections (from once-daily Copaxone to once-weekly Avonex), which side effects are more acceptable, and how well you feel on a specific drug.

The chief advantage of the injectable medications is that they're very safe. The side effects are known and there haven't been any unpleasant surprises after people have been on the drugs for years (or decades in some cases). Unfortunately, that doesn't mean they're easy to take. The side effects you have in the beginning often don't improve much over time. Flu-like symptoms can persist for years, wearing away at you with aches and pains and the feeling that you're coming down with something. Also unpleasant are the injection site reactions, which often don't get better with time.[11] With Copaxone, the skin denting and pitting caused by the injections are unsightly and may well be irreversible.

Of course the biggest drawback with the injectables is the injections themselves, and many studies over the years have shown to no one's great surprise that people don't like needles. In the very first MS treatment trial, most people stopped therapy within the first five years – despite having no other treatment available for their disease.[12] Many people tire of injections within a few months and up to one-half stop therapy within a few years.[13-16] Side effects are a common reason for stopping in the early days of treatment; later on, people often give up if they feel the medication isn't working.[17] An unfortunate consequence is that a first brush with an MS treatment is a turn-off for many: about one-third of people who go off their medication end up stopping therapy altogether.[18] That may change now that oral medications provide an alternative.

Physicians often speak of a drug's tolerability when referring to side effects. But the ability to tolerate something will be heavily determined by a person's accounting of whether the effort is worth it. Even nuisance effects will be intolerable if you feel that a medication isn't doing any good. If you're taking an injectable, you're able to manage the injections well enough and you feel the medication is doing some good, then by all means continue taking it. The one tautological take-home message from the long-term studies of injectables is: these medications do appear to produce a response in those people who respond. But for those who don't respond or who can't imagine injecting themselves regularly, the newer oral treatments are probably a better option.

OVER THE NEXT FEW YEARS, it's likely that oral and infusion drugs will eclipse the injectables and become the most popular MS therapies.[19,20] In comparing the injectables with the oral therapies, Aubagio appears to be about as effective as Rebif,[21] andTecfidera is about the same as Copaxone.[22] So either Tecfidera or Aubagio would certainly be a reasonable initial choice if you want to start with an oral medication. Both are good alternatives to injectable drugs.

Tecfidera can be a tough sell because of nausea/vomiting and stomach pain, especially in the first few months of treatment. But if you can handle those problems, the drug is likely to be effective in most cases.

Aubagio appears to be much easier to take. For women who are planning to become pregnant in the near future, Aubagio isn't the best choice because the drug persists so long in the body. It won't be enough simply to stop the medication if you are taking steps to become pregnant (or become pregnant). You will need to take cholestyramine or activated charcoal for 11 days to actively remove the drug from your body. This may be a bit unpleasant, but isn't an especially difficult or onerous requirement.

WHEN COMPARING DIFFERENT MEDICATIONS, one of the more important considerations is a drug's effectiveness. This factors in not only the efficacy seen in trials, but a person's ability and willingness to take the medication. This is one of the greatest problems faced by the injectables – people don't like taking them, so whatever efficacy they may have is hampered by their poor effectiveness in the real world. So in your assessment of your treatment options, don't neglect your personal preferences. Would you like an injectable or an oral medication? What are the side effects you think you can live with? And how well do you think you'll be able to continue taking that particular medication over the longer term?

Starting a treatment requires a commitment. Any medication needs to be taken as often as prescribed so it'll have a reasonable chance of working. So try it for three months or so. Typically your doctor will book an appointment to check on your progress within the first few months, and that's the best time to let your doctor or MS nurse know if you're having difficulties with the drug. It will be too early to tell if the drug is working, so the main goal will be to talk about side effects or any other problems you're having. In many cases, your doctor or nurse can give you tips to minimize the side effects. Of course you should keep your doctors informed about relapses, side effects or any other problems throughout the course of treatment, not just at your scheduled appointments.

If you can't live with the side effects or you think the drug is causing a worrisome new symptom, schedule an appointment as soon as possible. A drug that can't be tolerated is a treatment that has failed – so don't be shy about telling your doctor if you've stopped taking your medication (ideally you would tell them before stopping the drug on your own). If the initial choice of therapy hasn't worked out, keep in mind that you haven't failed the regimen, nor will you disappoint your doctor if you want to stop taking that particular drug. The medication has come up short, so you and your doctor will need to figure out Plan B as soon as possible.

If you can live with the side effects during the first few months, keep taking it regularly. You will also need to go for the various tests that are required to ensure that any problems (even if there are no symptoms) are caught early. After 6-9-months, it'll be time for you and your doctor to evaluate whether the treatment is working. The scheduling of appointments will depend on your clinic, but you'll certainly need to be re-examined within the first year of treatment. You should also have an MRI at this time to see if there's ongoing inflammation in the brain, although some centres are not always diligent in scheduling MRIs.

It isn't critical if the first choice of treatment isn't the best one. It's impossible to know ahead of time if a medication will be effective and whether you can live with the side effects. Each medication has a "personality". You may be put off at the beginning and want to try something else. You may get along well initially, but the relationship starts to sour. Keeping to the program can be difficult. Your medication doesn't have to be your new best friend, but you will have to live with it for a while. So if there's a problem with the drug – either it doesn't seem to be working or you can't handle the side effects – then you and your neurologist need to re-visit the original treatment decision. You do have other options. If you and your doctor feel your drug isn't a good match for you, it may be time to switch to the next medication. This is a matter of some urgency since treatments are likely to have a diminishing impact over time. If you're going to comparison shop, it's best to do that within the first few years after being diagnosed.

How do I know if my treatment isn't working?

THE USUAL MEASURING STICKS for a drug's effectiveness are its effects on relapses, MRI and disability scores. The most obvious sign that a treatment isn't working is if you continue to have relapses. One mild relapse (perhaps some numbness or tingling) may not be a reason to change therapies, especially in the first few months of starting a drug.[23] But after that, even one relapse may be too many,[24] especially if it's severe or the symptoms are new (e.g. bladder problems you didn't have before) or worrisome to you (e.g. difficulty walking or vertigo). During the injectable era it wasn't uncommon to have relapses – but that's less acceptable now that there are more effective alternatives. Expectations about treatment benefits were very modest during the injectable era, but the advent of second-generation medications has raised the bar about how effective a drug should be.

After a year on a treatment it's best to have an MRI. This is because there may be ongoing inflammatory activity in the brain – even if you're not having any relapses. A medication should suppress this inflammation. If it doesn't, there's a much higher risk of worsening MS. Some studies have found that the chance of relapsing over the next few years is up to eight times higher if there are any new lesions on an MRI.[25,26] More importantly, the presence of even one new inflammatory lesion means that your risk of disability progression over the next few years is 10-fold higher;[27,28] with two lesions, that risk may be 20-fold higher.[27]

Some inflammation is probably not avoidable in many people. With the so-called high-efficacy medications (Gilenya, Tysabri and Lemtrada), about 30% or so had a relapse in the first two years of treatment, and many had at least one new MRI lesion.[29-32] But better control of the inflammation in your brain and spinal cord will likely mean a better outcome in the future. If there are more than two or three new lesions,[24,33] this is strong evidence that your medication isn't working very well and it's time to think about changing to another therapy.

Another clue that a treatment isn't working is if you're showing signs of disability progression, which is usually evaluated with the EDSS scale. This needs to be assessed by a skilled physician every 6-12 months. One of the difficulties is that you may lose some function during or after a relapse, and the recovery period can be very lengthy (months or years). This loss of function is more of a worsening of your clinical status than actual progression of MS, but it may be a warning sign that a better treatment is needed. Unfortunately, neurologists may not regularly evaluate your EDSS score, preferring to rely on their own impressions of your clinical status. If an EDSS isn't done, you can track how well you're doing using the Patient Determined Disease Steps (PDDS) scale produced by the North American Research Consortium on Multiple Sclerosis (NARCOMS) group (the website is listed in the references).[34] Although the EDSS is often seen as being very complicated to administer, a person's rating of his/her own disability on the PDDS has been shown to match very closely to a neurologist's assessment using the EDSS.[35]

What is Plan B?

THE MEDICATION PLAN we've discussed thus far is for people who appear to have "mild" MS at the outset. So less potent medications (the injectables, Aubagio and Tecfidera) are often the initial choice for these people. This may be overly optimistic. Most people with MS – even those with mild disease – will develop disabilities during their lifetime. But by the time this worsening develops, it may be too late for the next medication to do much good.

This brings us to Plan B – starting one of the more potent medications (Gilenya, Tysabri and Lemtrada). These treatments are appropriate in three situations: 1) If a person has severe or high-risk MS at the outset, such as frequent, severe or worrisome symptoms, or risk factors for progressive disability (e.g. male, African-American); 2) if CNS inflammation (relapses, MRI lesions) is a persistent problem despite treatment with an injectable, Aubagio or Tecfidera (assuming you've been taking your treatment as directed); or 3) if you believe in the "chemotherapy" approach to MS – hitting the disease hard at the beginning to get the maximal benefit early on in the hope that this will mean less disability over the long term (see Chapter 11).

Some people, especially those who quit taking a drug, may shuttle from one of the less potent MS medications to another – from an interferon to Copaxone to Aubagio to Tecfidera. But arguably this is a waste of precious time. There is little sense in switching from one injectable to another, or from one first-line drug to another. As previously mentioned, the first five years of treatment are probably the most critical to the long-term outlook. So it may not be advisable to spend too much time test driving all of the first-choice therapies if there are more effective treatments that are more likely to get you where you need to go.

Does switching medications actually work?

YOU MAY THINK that if your MS doesn't respond well to one medication then it won't respond to another, but this isn't necessarily the case. The relapsing-remitting form of MS will respond to different treatments to a greater or lesser degree. (One day we hope the same can be said for progressive MS.) It's akin to having a bad headache that doesn't get any better with Tylenol. You may get some relief if you switch to Motrin/Advil or some other pain killer. This doesn't mean you illness is "drug-resistant". It's more a matter of individuals, with their unique physiology and unique ways of processing drugs, responding differently to a given medication.

It's fairly well established that a person who doesn't do that well on one medication can do better if they switch treatments. Many of these studies have looked at switching from one injectable to another, but it's less likely that people will do this now that oral therapies are available.

The more likely scenarios are switching from an interferon or Copaxone to an oral therapy such as Aubagio or Tecfidera, or switching from either interferon/Copaxone or Aubagio/Tecfidera to a more potent therapy such as Gilenya, Tysabri or Lemtrada.

In the clinical trials of Aubagio and Tecfidera, the drugs appeared to be somewhat more effective in newly-diagnosed people compared to those who were coming off a previous treatment (i.e. had switched from another drug),[36,37] although this is generally true of all the MS medications. This is likely because previously-treated people are a selected group with more active disease. However, both drugs did reduce relapses in these people, so they were having an effect.

No studies have looked at switching from first-line Aubagio or Tecfidera to a second-line drug. But one consideration is whether a given treatment will affect later decisions down the road. If you switch from Aubagio to a drug with immunosuppressant effects (such as Tysabri and possibly Gilenya), it would probably be best to undergo the active elimination protocol to remove Aubagio from your system beforehand. If you start with Tecfidera, there's a potential risk of PML (one case of PML has occurred with Tecfidera), so it may not be a good idea to switch to Tysabri. The PML risk with Tysabri hasn't been broken down according to what treatment people were taking before, so it isn't known if prior treatment with Aubagio or Tecfidera (or Gilenya for that matter) will alter the PML risk once you're on Tysabri. This uncertainty – just one of several – is another reason why it's probably best to stop Tysabri after two years (24 doses).

SOMEWHAT MORE IS KNOWN about going from an injectable to either Tysabri or Gilenya. There have been several reports of good success rates when switching from an injectable to Tysabri. In one such study, relapses were reduced by three-quarters;[38] in another, about 85% of people had no relapses at all in the year after starting Tysabri.[39] A third study found that people were more likely to keep taking Tysabri rather than an injectable,[40] which may be because they felt much better (or because their dose-taking was being supervised at an infusion centre).

One of the pivotal trials of Gilenya (called TRANSFORMS) directly compared it with Avonex and found that Gilenya was the more effective therapy.[41] This appeared to be confirmed when people on Avonex later switched to Gilenya and did much better.[42] Other Gilenya studies have also shown that relapse rates go down over 50%,[43] people are much less likely to stop treatment,[44] and that they're more satisfied with their therapy.[45-47]

So these findings are consistent with what's known about Tysabri and Gilenya. Both appear to be more effective than the injectables, and both appear to give an added boost to reducing relapses and MRI activity.

Lemtrada is generally accepted as the most potent therapy. However, it's the newest drug on the market and hasn't been studied as extensively as other MS medications. Lemtrada was significantly more effective than Rebif in both CARE-MS studies.[31,32] In CARE-MS II, over 70% of people had been on another therapy,[32] so switching from an injectable to Lemtrada appears to be safe. Only 3% of people were previously treated with Tysabri and none had received an oral before switching to Lemtrada, so not enough is known about these switches.

How do I choose a higher potency drug?

IF YOU DON'T DO WELL ENOUGH on a first-choice medication, it may be time to consider starting a more potent medication, such as Tysabri, Gilenya or Lemtrada. (This assumes that you don't live in a country where people have the option of starting with one of these drugs right away.)

Which of these is better?

No clinical trials have directly compared these three medications. One study estimated that people who switched either to Tysabri or Gilenya would do equally well.[48] In part, how well the person does will depend on how active their disease is at the time of switching.

Another way of comparing the effectiveness of the different treatments is by looking at the so-called disease activity-free rates (DAF) – an important emerging topic in MS. A sign of its emergence is the variety of terms used to describe it, such as NEDA (no evidence of disease activity), NEIDA (no evidence of inflammatory disease activity), among others. All of these terms refer to the idea of having no relapses, no new MRI activity, and no short-term disability progression with a treatment. Relapses and MRI refer to the inflammatory component of MS. Progression as assessed by the EDSS scale is the outlier: it's more a measure of cumulative processes that contribute to neurodegenerative changes; it's difficult to evaluate probably; and the way it's usually measured (a change in EDSS score that persists for three or six months) isn't very accurate.

It's important to note that "free of disease activity" doesn't mean "free of disease" (although this measure is sometimes erroneously called "disease-free"). If you look hard enough, you will find evidence of disease activity. So really NEDA (now the preferred term) is primarily useful as a way of comparing the impact of different medications.

As you might expect, the best NEDA results have been seen with Tysabri, Gilenya and Lemtrada. After one year, 47% of people on Tysabri were disease activity-free,[49] 46% with Gilenya,[50] and 44% on Lemtrada.[51] But the results after two years are a better measure of long-term effectiveness: 37% with Tysabri,[49] 33% with Gilenya,[52] and 32-39% with Lemtrada.[31,32]

In choosing among the high-potency medications, it's best to review the earlier chapters about these drugs to get a sense of their effectiveness and side effects. All have potentially serious side effects, but we'll see if we can put these into a broader context.

Gilenya is available as a first-choice drug in some countries, and an argument could be made that it's a suitable option soon after diagnosis to shut down inflammation more effectively. However, the general recommendation is to use it as a back-up when another drug fails unless the person has especially active disease at the outset.[24,53,54] The biggest concern with Gilenya is its effects on the heart. There's a small risk of heart-rhythm disturbances, so it's not the best choice for people with established heart disease. Individuals with diabetes may be at risk of developing eye problems, although this hasn't been well studied. The biggest nuisance is the hassle of starting the drug. For the first dose, you'll need to be kept under observation at the clinic for six hours (bring a book) and undergo heart monitoring (pulse, blood pressure and ECG). Some people will experience a slowing in their heart rate, which can cause symptoms such as dizziness. A slow walk around the observation room is often enough to keep the heart rate up. The six-hour observation period will be off-putting to some, but afterward the once-a-day capsule is easy enough to take and serious side effects aren't that common.[55,56]

Tysabri is usually not a first option. It's generally very well tolerated,[57] but its use should probably be limited to two years' duration. Of course the main concern with Tysabri is the risk of PML. Being tested for JC virus antibodies every six months is used to flag an increasing risk of PML, although this wasn't the original intent of the test. Testing is one component of an overall "risk management plan", but arguably that plan has not been very successful. The risk of developing PML is now higher than when the plan was first started.[58,59] For a given individual, the risk of PML is certainly low in the first two years of treatment. Beyond that, the risk hasn't been quantified and long-term treatment isn't something that should be encouraged.

There is a broader concern as well. The number of PML cases has climbed rapidly, with over 100 new cases per years. One in five people who develop PML will die; many of the remaining will have profound disability. With other treatments on the market – Gilenya and Lemtrada, as well as other high-potency drugs in development – it may well be that Tysabri will be viewed as a poor option in the future. Indeed, what will regulators think when there are 600 cases of PML (expected in 2015), or 1,000? There have been over 100 PML deaths thus far with Tysabri. Will the FDA intervene when there are 150 deaths, or 200? Unless more can be learned about how PML develops, Tysabri's future may be limited as an MS therapy.

A further difficulty with Tysabri is stopping the drug, in part because of the way it works. Tysabri isn't a true immunomodulatory agent. It doesn't alter the immune response. Rather, it blocks activated T cells from getting into the CNS. This is a good strategy for reducing inflammation in the brain – as shown by the efficacy data in clinical trials – but it also means that the activated T cells remain activated. There have even been some suggestions that Tysabri can worsen inflammation,[60,61] but this doesn't translate into worsening MS because the barrier is up. These activated T cells are the "barbarians at the gate". If Tysabri is stopped and the gates fall, there's an angry mob of T cells ready to rush in. What this means is that when you stop taking Tysabri, as the drug leaches out of your system (which takes a few months), there's a very real risk that your MS will get worse. How much worse is a matter of debate, but it's quite likely that any gains you make while on Tysabri will be lost within a few months of stopping the drug.[62]

The problem is that this renewed disease activity is hard to shut down. Many people find that their MS flares up despite going onto another treatment, such as steroids, an interferon, Copaxone or even an immunosuppressant.[63-65] Gilenya appears to be somewhat effective treatment for controlling post-Tysabri flare-ups – assuming you haven't already tried Gilenya before – but it works best if you start it within a month or two of stopping Tysabri.[66,67] Lemtrada may be more effective after Tysabri, but the drug takes a while before it becomes fully active, and the safety of this approach haven't been studied.

Where Lemtrada will fit into the treatment plan has not yet been fully worked out. The most obvious uses will be in people with severe disease from the outset, and those who haven't responded well enough to one or more medications. The temptation will be to keep it in reserve as a treatment of last resort, but this may not be the best use of this drug. It may be better to use it earlier in an "induction" approach – hitting MS hard to knock out the disease process. Once the disease process is under control, a person could continue with annual courses of Lemtrada or switch to another, less potent medication over the longer term to try to maintain the gains that have been made. This latter strategy hasn't been formally studied yet, but has been the subject of discussion at scientific meetings,[68] and it's likely to receive more attention in the years ahead.

So the general plan for MS treatment is to start with the drug that will adequately control your symptoms. In many cases, this will be Aubagio or Tecfidera. If your MS is more severe, an early switch to Gilenya or Lemtrada may be a good idea. The general preference may be for one of these higher potency drugs rather than Tysabri, both to avoid the higher risk of PML and to sidestep the problems involved in stopping Tysabri. This is simply a common-sense suggestion: why start a drug that you'll have to stop within a couple of years?

Is treatment safe?

ALL MEDICATIONS CAN CAUSE SIDE EFFECTS. All medications have the potential to do more harm than good. But we accept the idea of some degree of risk every time we take an Aspirin, a birth control pill, an antihistamine, or an antacid. So starting an MS medication isn't a question of whether there will be a risk. The questions that people need to ask themselves are: Is the risk too great for the benefits I'll receive; and Am I prepared to take on that risk?

When looking at risks, the things to consider are the type of risk, the likelihood of it happening, and if you can accept that risk if it happens to you. Part of this assessment will be based on facts – numbers and statistics. But equally important is the part that's entirely subjective. For example, the flu-like symptoms that are a routine part of taking an interferon are not serious in themselves. To many they may seem like a small price to pay – at first. But feeling as if you're coming down with the flu proved to be a common reason why people stopped taking the drug. Similarly, many will experience flushing or nausea when they start Tecfidera. You may be able to put up with that for a period of time, and perhaps these nuisance symptoms will get better within a couple of months. Or you may feel that these symptoms are more intrusive than your MS symptoms, and decide you're better off without them.

Some side effects are potentially more serious, and you'll want to reassure yourself that they can be detected early and managed if they do occur. An example is liver damage. The liver is where many medications are broken down, so it's on the front line of drug exposure and very susceptible to injury. Fortunately, there are early warning signs of liver damage (e.g. changes in liver enzyme levels) that can be detected with periodic blood tests. If damage is occurring, lowering the dose or stopping the drug altogether can allow the liver to heal itself before the problem becomes irreversible. So potential liver problems are fairly manageable if you go regularly to get a blood test.

With the bigger guns, the concerns are potentially bigger. With Gilenya, some testing will have to be done in advance to avoid some risks. For example, your doctor needs to ensure that you've been exposed to the chickenpox virus before you take the drug. If you haven't been exposed, you'll need a vaccination before starting treatment. A bigger concern with Gilenya is its possible effects on the heart, which is why you need to be under observation by trained medical staff when you start the drug. In most cases, these heart effects aren't noticeable to the person. The tests that are performed (ECG, pulse, blood pressure) can identify if there's a problem even if you don't detect anything. Significant problems are rare, and Gilenya appears to have minimal effects on heart function after a couple of weeks. The other potential side effect with Gilenya that needs to be managed is eye problems. After 3-4 months on treatment, you'll need an eye exam because the drug can affect vision in about one in 300 people.[69] A second exam may be advisable a year later since eye changes can occur later on,[69] and you'll want to ensure that a problem isn't developing.

The main concerns with Tysabri are early and late effects. Some people react badly to the infusion, so you'll need to remain under observation for about an hour after taking the drug. The other problem, of course, is PML. The risk of developing PML increases over time and starts becoming worrisome in a year or two (although some people have developed PML more quickly than that). Because the consequences of PML are so devastating, it's often best to stop taking Tysabri – no matter how well you feel – after two years on the drug.

Lemtrada can be difficult to start because most will react to the infusion (headache, rash, nausea and fever), although a course of steroids will help. About one in six people will develop thyroid problems, skin reactions are common, and most people will be susceptible to different types of infection. Serious side effects, such as bleeding complications, are uncommon (about 1%). The biggest nuisance is the need for monthly blood tests during the course of treatment.

Looking to the future

THE WORLD OF MS CHANGED two decades ago when the first of the disease-modifying therapies was introduced. Before that, doctors were often reluctant to diagnose MS because the prognosis was poor and nothing could be done. MS was about uncertainty and waiting: for symptoms to appear, for disability to show itself. The practice of watchful waiting was deeply ingrained, and ten years would pass after the first MS treatment was studied before there was a general consensus that therapy was worthwhile and should be started as soon as possible.

It is still too early to say how much disease-modifying therapies actually modify the course of the disease, but the general impression is that people are much better off now. Part of that can be attributed to earlier diagnosis, but much of it is likely due to treatments dampening the inflammatory flare-ups that are so damaging to the delicate tissues of the brain and spinal cord.

Given the wealth of treatment choices now available, it might seem improbable that some would prefer to remain untreated, but this is so. The reasons for this are as individual as the people themselves. Some are skeptical about medications in general, believe their doctors are simply pushing drugs at the behest of pharmaceutical companies, or would prefer to try alternative therapies. Some try to put the reality of their MS out of their minds, and may be falsely reassured when their symptoms go away for a time. The more consumer-minded may question the wisdom of medications that may make you feel worse – isn't a product supposed to make you feel better?

You can certainly question the benefits of any or all of the medications, and you may feel that you're better off with the MS you know rather than the drugs and side effects you don't know. That is your right. But the hard fact is that MS is likely to become very disabling in a decade or two. It isn't a sure bet that treating it today will make things better later on. But it's a certainty that not treating it will allow MS to run its course unchecked, and the consequences will be what they will be. Starting a treatment today may save you from the future regret that you didn't do everything possible when you could.

There are many difficult decisions to make when you are first diagnosed with MS, and more hard choices – about your family, your career, about coping with your illness – as life unfolds. At each decision point you will have a choice. Consult those around you – your doctors, partner, family and friends. Make sure you have all the information you need. The goal of *Treating Your MS* is not to advocate one treatment over another or to dictate what must be done. That decision is yours. But the sincere hope is that explaining the details of what's known about MS and the medications used to treat it will enable you to make more fully informed decisions about how best to live with your MS.

References

CHAPTER 1. WHAT IS MS?

1. Mayo L, Quintana FJ, Weiner HL. The innate immune system in demyelinating disease. Immunol Rev 2012;248:170-87.

2. Krone B, Oeffner F, Grange JM. Is the risk of multiple sclerosis related to the 'biography' of the immune system? J Neurol 2009;256:1052-60.

3. Rawji KS, Yong VW. The benefits and detriments of macrophages/microglia in models of multiple sclerosis. Clin Dev Immunol 2013;2013:948976.

4. Skripuletz T, Hackstette D, Bauer K, et al. Astrocytes regulate myelin clearance through recruitment of microglia during cuprizone-induced demyelination. Brain 2013;136(Pt 1):147-67.

5. Kurtzke JF. Epidemiologic evidence for multiple sclerosis as an infection. Clin Microbiol Rev 1993;6:382-427.

6. Sospedra M, Martin R. Molecular mimicry in multiple sclerosis. Autoimmunity 2006;39:3-8.

7. Fujinami RS, Oldstone MB. Molecular mimicry as a mechanism for virus-induced autoimmunity. Immunol Res 1989;8:3-15.

8. Sumaya CV, Myers LW, Ellison GW. Epstein-Barr virus antibodies in multiple sclerosis. Arch Neurol 1980;37:94-6.

9. Larsen PD, Bloomer LC, Bray PF. Epstein-Barr nuclear antigen and viral capsid antigen antibody titers in multiple sclerosis. Neurology 1985;35:435-8.

10. Warner HB, Carp RI. Multiple sclerosis etiology – an Epstein-Barr virus hypothesis. Med Hypotheses 1988;25:93-7.

11. Haahr S, Sommerlund M, Møller-Larsen A, et al. Is multiple sclerosis caused by a dual infection with retrovirus and Epstein-Barr virus? Neuroepidemiology 1992;11:299-303.

12. Nowak J, Januszkiewicz D, Pernak M, et al. Multiple sclerosis-associated virus-related pol sequences found both in multiple sclerosis and healthy donors are more frequently expressed in multiple sclerosis patients. J Neurovirol 2003;9:112-7.

13. Nielsen TR, Rostgaard K, Nielsen NM, et al. Multiple sclerosis after infectious mononucleosis. Arch Neurol 2007;64:72-5.

14. Hernán MA, Zhang SM, Lipworth L, et al. Multiple sclerosis and age at infection with common viruses. Epidemiology 2001;12:301-6.

15. Ascherio A, Munger KL, Lennette ET, et al. Epstein-Barr virus antibodies and risk of multiple sclerosis: a prospective study. JAMA 2001;286:3083-8.

16. Myhr KM, Riise T, Barrett-Connor E, et al. Altered antibody pattern to Epstein-Barr virus but not to other herpesviruses in multiple sclerosis: a population based case-control study from western Norway. J Neurol Neurosurg Psychiatry 1998;64:539-42.

17. Lehmann PV, Forsthuber T, Miller A, et al. Spreading of T-cell autoimmunity to cryptic determinants of an autoantigen. Nature 1992; 558:155-7.

18. Katz-Levy Y, Neville KL, Girvin AM, et al. Endogenous presentation of self myelin epitopes by CNS-resident APCs in Theiler's virus-infected mice. J Clin Invest 1999;104:599-610.

19. Wandinger K, Jabs W, Siekhaus A, et al. Association between clinical disease activity and Epstein-Barr virus reactivation in MS. Neurology 2000;55:178-84.

20. Lycke J, Svennerholm B, Hjelmquist E, et al. Acyclovir treatment of relapsing-remitting multiple sclerosis. A randomized, placebo-controlled, double-blind study. J Neurol 1996;243:214-24.

21. Bech E, Lycke J, Gadeberg P, et al. A randomized, double-blind, placebo-controlled MRI study of anti-herpes virus therapy in MS. Neurology 2002;58:31-6.

22. Friedman JE, Zabriskie JB, Plank C, et al. A randomized clinical trial of valacyclovir in multiple sclerosis. Mult Scler 2005;11:286-95.

23. Allen M, Sandberg-Wollheim M, Sjogren K, et al. Association of susceptibility to multiple sclerosis in Sweden with HLA class II DRB1 and DQB1 alleles. Hum Immunol 1994;39:41-8.

24. Masterman T, Ligers A, Olsson T, et al. HLA-DR15 is associated with lower age at onset in multiple sclerosis. Ann Neurol 2000;48:211-9.

25. Handunnetthi L, Ramagopalan SV, Ebers GC. Multiple sclerosis, vitamin D, and *HLA-DRB1*15*. Neurology 2010;74:1905-10.

26. Amirzargar A, Mytilineos J, Yousefipour A, et al. HLA class II (DRB1, DQA1 and DQB1) associated genetic susceptibility in Iranian multiple sclerosis (MS) patients. Eur J Immunogenet 1998;25:297-301.

27. Brassat D, Salemi G, Barcellos LF, et al. The HLA locus and multiple sclerosis in Sicily. Neurology 2005;64:361-3.

28. Quelvennec E, Bera O, Cabre P, et al. Genetic and functional studies in multiple sclerosis patients from Martinique attest for a specific and direct role of the HLA-DR locus in the syndrome. Tissue Antigens 2003;61:166-71.

29. Oksenberg JR, Barcellos LF, Cree BA, et al. Mapping multiple sclerosis susceptibility to the HLA-DR locus in African Americans. Am J Hum Genet 2004;74:160-7.

30. Rojas OL, Rojas-Villarraga A, Cruz-Tapias P, et al. HLA class II polymorphism in Latin American patients with multiple sclerosis. Autoimmun Rev 2010;9:407-13.

31. Dyment DA, Sadnovich AD, Ebers GC. Genetics of multiple sclerosis. Hum Mol Genet 1997;6:1693-8.

32. Waubant E, Mowry EM, Krupp L, et al. Antibody response to common viruses and human leukocyte antigen-DRB1 in pediatric multiple sclerosis. Mult Scler 2012;19:891-5.

33. Fleming JO, Cook TD. Multiple sclerosis and the hygiene hypothesis. Neurology 2006;67:2085-6.

34. Ponsonby AL, van der Mei I, Dwyer T, et al. Exposure to infant siblings during early life and risk of multiple sclerosis. JAMA 2005;293:463-9.

35. Conradi S, Malzahn U, Schröter F, et al. Environmental factors in early childhood are associated with multiple sclerosis: a case-control study. BMC Neurol 2011;11:123.

36. Levin LI, Munger KL, Rubertone MV, et al. Temporal relationship between elevation of epstein-barr virus antibody titers and initial onset of neurological symptoms in multiple sclerosis. JAMA 2005;293:2496-500.

37. Sundström P, Juto P, Wadell G, et al. An altered immune response to Epstein-Barr virus in multiple sclerosis: a prospective study.Neurology 2004;62:2277-82.

38. World map of prevalence of multiple sclerosis. www.mult-sclerosis.org/ms_world.html.

39. Beretich BD, Beretich TM. Explaining multiple sclerosis prevalence by ultraviolet exposure: a geospatial analysis. Mult Scler 2009;15: 891-8.

40. Pierrot-Deseilligny P, Souberbielle J-C. Is hypovitaminosis D one of the environmental risk factors for multiple sclerosis? Brain 2010:133;1869-88.

41. Sadovnick AD, Duquette P, Herrera B, et al. A timing-of-birth effect on multiple sclerosis clinical phenotype. Neurology 2007;69:60-2.

42. Willer CJ, Dyment DA, Sadovnick AD, et al. Timing of birth and risk of multiple sclerosis: population based study. Br Med J 2005;330:120-4.

43. Fiddes B, Wason J, Kemppinen A, et al. Confounding rather than biology underlies the apparent association between month of birth and multiple sclerosis. Ann Neurol 2013;73:714-20.

44. Acheson ED, Bachrach CA, Wright FM. Some comments on the relationship of the distribution of multiple sclerosis to latitude, solar radiation, and other variables. Acta Psychiatr Scand Suppl 1960;35:132-47.

45. Goldberg P, Fleming MC, Picard EH. Multiple sclerosis: decreased relapse rate through dietary supplementation with calcium, magnesium and vitamin D. Med Hypotheses 1986;21:193-200.

46. Muller K, Bendtzen K. Inhibition of human T lymphocyte proliferation and cytokine production by 1,25-dihydroxyvitamin D3. Differential effects on CD45RA+ and CD45R0+ cells. Autoimmunity 1992;14:37-43.

47. Cantorna MT, Hayes CE, DeLuca HF. 1,25-Dihydroxyvitamin D3 reversibly blocks the progression of relapsing encephalomyelitis, a model of multiple sclerosis. Proc Natl Acad Sci USA 1996;93:7861-4.

48. Bhalla AK, Amento EP, Clemens TL, et al. Specific high affinity receptors for 1,25-dihydroxyvitamin D3 in human peripheral blood mononuclear cells: presence in monocytes and induction in T lymphocytes following activation. J Clin Endocrinol Metab 1983;57:1308-10.

49. Vedman CM, Cantorna MT, DeLuca HF. Expression of 1,25-dihydroxyvitamin D(3) receptor in the immune system. Arch Biochem Biophys 2000;374:334-8.

50. Chen S, Sims GP, Chen XX, Gu YY, Chen S, Lipsky PE. Modulatory effect of 1,25-dihydroxyvitamin D3 on human B cell differentiation. J Immunol 2007;179:1634-47.

51. Hayes CE, Nashold FE, Spach KM, et al. The immunological functions of the vitamin D endocrine system. Cell Mol Biol (Noisy-le-grand) 2003;49:277-300.

52. Stein MS, Liu Y, Gray OM, et al. A randomized trial of high-dose vitamin D2 in relapsing-remitting multiple sclerosis. Neurology 2011;77:1611-8.

53. Houghton LA, Veith R. The case against ergocalciferol (vitamin D2) as a vitamin supplement. Am J Clin Nutr 2006;84:694-7.

54. Mosayebi G, Ghazavi A, Ghasami K, et al. Therapeutic effect of vitamin D3 in multiple sclerosis patients. Immunol Invest 2011;40:627-39.

CHAPTER 2. HOW DOES MS DEVELOP?

1. McDonald WI, Compston A, Edan G, et al. Recommended diagnostic criteria for multiple sclerosis: guidelines from the international panel on the diagnosis of multiple sclerosis. Ann Neurol 2001;50:121-7.

2. Polman CH, Reingold SC, Edan G, et al. Diagnostic criteria for multiple sclerosis: 2005 revisions to the "McDonald Criteria". Ann Neurol 2005;58:840-6.

3. Polman CH, Reingold SC, Banwell B, et al. Diagnostic criteria for multiple sclerosis: 2010 revisions to the McDonald Criteria. Ann Neurol 2011;69:292-302.

4. Okuda DT, Mowry EM, Beheshtian A, et al. Incidental MRI anomalies suggestive of multiple sclerosis: the radiologically isolated syndrome. Neurology 2009;72:800-5.

5. Morrissey SP, Miller DH, Kendall BE, et al. The significance of brain magnetic resonance imaging abnormalities at presentation with clinically isolated syndromes suggestive of multiple sclerosis. A 5-year follow-up study. Brain 1993;116(Pt 1):135-46.

6. O'Riordan JI, Thompson AJ, Kingsley DP, et al. The prognostic value of brain MRI in clinically isolated syndromes of the CNS. A 10-year follow-up. Brain 1998;121(Pt 3):495-503.

7. Optic Neuritis Study Group. Multiple sclerosis risk after optic neuritis: final Optic Neuritis Treatment Trial follow-up. Arch Neurol 2008;65:727-32.

8. Young J, Quinn S, Hurrell M, et al. Clinically isolated acute transverse myelitis: prognostic features and incidence. Mult Scler 2009;15:1295-302.

9. Sastre-Garriga J, Tintore M, Rovira A, et al. Conversion to multiple sclerosis after a clinically isolated syndrome of the brainstem: cranial magnetic resonance imaging, cerebrospinal fluid and neurophysiological findings. Mult Scler 2003;9:39-43.

10. Morrow SA, Fraser JA, Nicolle D, et al. Predicting conversion to MS – the role of a history suggestive of demyelination. Can J Neurol Sci 2010;37:488-91.

11. Kelly SB, Chaila E, Kinsella K, et al. Using atypical symptoms and red flags to identify non-demyelinating disease. J Neurol Neurosurg Psychiatry 2012;83:44-8.

12. Brex PA, Miszkiel KA, O'Riordan JI, et al. Assessing the risk of early multiple sclerosis in patients with clinically isolated syndromes: the role of a follow up MRI. J Neurol Neurosurg Psychiatry 2001;70:390-3.

13. Uitdehaag BMJ, Kappos L, Bauer L, et al. Discrepancies in the interpretation of clinical symptoms and signs in the diagnosis of multiple sclerosis. A proposal for standardization. Mult Scler 2005;11:227-31.

14. Nielsen JM1 Moraal B, Polman CH, et al. Classification of patients with a clinically isolated syndrome based on signs and symptoms is supported by magnetic resonance imaging results. Mult Scler 2007;13:717-21.

15. Mowry EM, Pesic M, Grimes B, et al. Clinical predictors of early second event in patients with clinically isolated syndrome. J Neurol 2009;256:1061-6.

16. Tortorella C, Bellacosa A, Paolicell D, et al. Age-related gadolinium-enhancement of MRI brain lesions in multiple sclerosis. J Neurol Sci 2005;239:95-9.

17. Filippi M, Wolinsky JS, Sormani MP, et al. Enhancement frequency decreases with increasing age in relapsing-remitting multiple sclerosis. Neurology 2001;56:422-3.

18. Dobson R, Ramagopalan S, Giovannoni G. The effect of gender in clinically isolated syndrome (CIS): a meta-analysis. Mult Scler 2012;18:600-4.

19. Jacobs LD, Beck RW, Simon JH, et al. Intramuscular interferon beta-1a therapy initiated during a first demyelinating event in multiple sclerosis. N Engl J Med 2000;343:898-904.

20. Comi G, Filippi M, Barkhof F, et al. Effect of early interferon treatment on conversion to definite multiple sclerosis: a randomised study. Lancet 2001;357:1576-82.

21. Comi G, De Stefano N, Freedman MS, et al. Comparison of two dosing frequencies of subcutaneous interferon beta-1a in patients with a first clinical demyelinating event suggestive of multiple sclerosis (REFLEX): a phase 3 randomised controlled trial. Lancet Neurol 2012;11:33-41.

22. Kappos L, Polman CH, Freedman MS, et al. Treatment with interferon beta-1b delays conversion to clinically definite and McDonald MS in patients with clinically isolated syndromes. Neurology 2006;67:1242-9.

23. Comi G, Martinelli V, Rodegher M, et al. Effect of glatiramer acetate on conversion to clinically definite multiple sclerosis in patients with clinically isolated syndrome (PreCISe study): a randomised, double-blind, placebo-controlled trial. Lancet 2009;374:1503-11.

24. Comi G, Martinelli V, Rodegher M, et al. Effects of early treatment with glatiramer acetate in patients with clinically isolated syndrome. Mult Scler 2012;19:1074-83.

25. Kinkel RP, Kollman C, O'Connor P, et al. IM interferon beta-1a delays definite multiple sclerosis 5 years after a first demyelinating event. Neurology 2006;66:678-84.

26. D'Alessandro R, Vignatelli L, Lugaresi A, et al. Risk of multiple sclerosis following clinically isolated syndrome: a 4-year prospective study. J Neurol 2013;260:1583-93.

27. Sormani MP, Tintore M, Rovaris M, et al. Will Rogers phenomenon in multiple sclerosis. Ann Neurol 2008;64:428-33.

28. Miller DH, Chard DT, Ciccarelli O. Clinically isolated syndromes. Lancet Neurol 2012;11:157-69.

29. Kappos L, Freedman MS, Polman CH, et al. Long-term effect of early treatment with interferon beta-1b after a first clinical event suggestive of multiple sclerosis: 5-year active treatment extension of the phase 3 BENEFIT trial. Lancet Neurol 2009;8:987-97.

30. Kinkel RP, Dontchew M, Kollman C, et al. Association between immediate initiation of intramuscular interferon beta-1a at the time of a clinically isolated syndrome and long-term outcomes: a 10-year follow-up of the Controlled High-Risk Avonex Multiple Sclerosis Prevention Study in Ongoing Neurological Surveillance. Arch Neurol 2012;69:183-90.

31. Feuillet L, Reuter F, Audoin B, et al. Early cognitive impairment in patients with clinically isolated syndrome suggestive of multiple sclerosis. Mult Scler 2007;13:124-7.

32. Summers M, Swanton J, Fernando K, et al. Cognitive impairment in multiple sclerosis can be predicted by imaging early in the disease. J Neurol Neurosurg Psychiatry 2008;79:955-8.

33. Khalil M, Enzinger C, Langhammer C, et al. Cognitive impairment in relation to MRI metrics in patients with clinically isolated syndrome. Mult Scler 2011;17:173-80.

34. Glanz BI, Healy BC, Hviid LE, et al. Cognitive deterioration in patients with early multiple sclerosis: a 5-year study. J Neurol Neurosurg Psychiatry 2012;83:38-43.

35. Penner IK, Stemper B, Calabrese P, et al. Effects of interferon beta-1b on cognitive performance in patients with a first event suggestive of multiple sclerosis. Mult Scler 2012;18:1466-71.

36. Miller A, Wolinsky J, Kappos L, et al. TOPIC main outcomes: efficacy and safety of once-daily oral teriflunomide in patients with clinically isolated syndrome. Presented at the 29th Congress of the European Committee for Treatment and Research in Multiple Sclerosis, Copenhagen, Denmark, October 2-5, 2013; abstract 99.

CHAPTER 3. WHAT CAN I EXPECT?

1. Lublin FD, Reingold SC. Defining the clinical course of multiple sclerosis: results of an international survey. National Multiple Sclerosis Society (USA) Advisory Committee on Clinical Trials of New Agents in Multiple Sclerosis. Neurology 1996;46:907-11.

2. Kremenchutzky M, Cottrell D, Rice G, et al. The natural history of multiple sclerosis: a geographically based study. 7. Progressive-relapsing and relapsing-progressive multiple sclerosis: a re-evaluation. Brain 1999;122(Pt 10):1941-50.

3. Confavreux C, Compston DA, Hommes OR, et al. EDMUS, a European database for multiple sclerosis. J Neurol Neurosurg Psychiatry 1992;55:671-6.

4. Confavreux C, Vukusic S, Moreau T, Adeleine P. Relapses and progression of disability in multiple sclerosis. N Engl J Med 2000;343:1430-8.

5. Kurtzke JF. Rating neurologic impairment in multiple sclerosis: an expanded disability status scale (EDSS). Neurology 1983;33:1444-52.

6. Scalfari A, Neuhaus A, Degenhardt A, et al. The natural history of multiple sclerosis, a geographically based study 10: relapses and long-term disability. Brain 2010;133:1914-29.

7. Tremlett H, Paty D, Devonshire V. Disability progression in multiple sclerosis is slower than previously reported. Neurology 2006;66:172-7.

8. Steinman L. Multiple sclerosis: a two-stage disease. Nat Immunol 2001;2:762-4.

9. Vollmer T. The natural history of relapses in multiple sclerosis. J Neurol Sci 2007; 256: S5-S13.

10. Confavreux C, Vukusic S. Natural history of multiple sclerosis: a unifying concept. Brain 2006;129:606-16.

11. Confavreux C, Vukusic S, Adeleine P. Early clinical predictors and progression of irreversible disability in multiple sclerosis: an amnesic process. Brain 2003;126:770-82.

12. Leray E, Yaouanq J, Le Page E, et al. Evidence for a two-stage disability progression in multiple sclerosis. Brain 2010:133;1900-13.

13. Pittock SJ, McClelland RL, Mayr WT, et al. Clinical implications of benign multiple sclerosis: a 20-year population-based follow-up study. Ann Neurol 2004;56:303-6.

14. Riise T, Gronning M, Fernández O, et al. Early prognostic factors for disability in multiple sclerosis, a European multicenter study. Acta Neurol Scand 1992;85:212-8.

15. Bergamaschi R, Berzuini C, Romani A, Cosi V. Predicting secondary progression in relapsing-remitting multiple sclerosis: a Bayesian analysis. J Neurol Sci 2001;189:13-21.

16. Leone MA, Bonissoni S, Collimedaglia L, et al. Factors predicting incomplete recovery from relapses in multiple sclerosis: a prospective study. Mult Scler 2008;14:485-93.

17. Runmarker B, Andersen O. Prognostic factors in a multiple sclerosis incidence cohort with twenty-five years of follow-up. Brain 1993;116(Pt 1):117-34.

18. Thygesen P. Evaluation of drug treatment of disseminated sclerosis. Ugeskr Laeger 1965; 127:1448-50.

19. Tremlett H, Zhao Y, Joseph J, Devonshire V, UBCMS Clinic Neurologists. Relapses in multiple sclerosis are age and time-dependent. J Neurol Neurosurg Psychiatry 2008;79:1368-74.

20. Scalfari A, Neuhaus A, Degenhardt A, et al. The natural history of multiple sclerosis, a geographically based study 10: relapses and long-term disability. Brain 2010; 133:1914-29.

21. Binquet C, Quantin C, Le Teuff G, Pagliano JF, Abrahamowicz M, Moreau T. The prognostic value of initial relapses on the evolution of disability in patients with relapsing-remitting multiple sclerosis. Neuroepidemiology 2006;27:45-54.

22. Bosca I, Coret F, Valero C, et al. Effect of relapses over early progression of disability in multiple sclerosis patients treated with beta-interferon. Mult Scler 2008;14:636-9.

23. Sormani MP, Rio J, Tintore M, et al. Scoring treatment response in patients with relapsing multiple sclerosis Mult Scler 2012;19:605-12.

24. Hirst CL, Ingram G, Pickersgill TP, Robertson NP. Temporal evolution of remission following multiple sclerosis relapse and predictors of outcome. Mult Scler 2012;18:1152-8.

25. Lublin FD, Reingold SC, Cohen JA, et al. Defining the clinical course of multiple sclerosis: the 2013 revisions. Neurology 2014;83:278-286.

26. Lublin FD, Baier M, Cutter G. Effect of relapses on development of residual deficit in multiple sclerosis. Neurology. 2003;61:1528-32.

27. Hirst C, Ingram G, Pearson O, Pickersgill T, Scolding N, Robertson N. Contribution of relapses to disability in multiple sclerosis. J Neurol 2008;255:280-7.

28. Cossburn M, Ingram G, Hirst C, et al. Age at onset as a determinant of presenting phenotype and initial relapse recovery in multiple sclerosis. Mult Scler 2012;18:45-54.

29. Vercellino M, Romagnolo A, Mattioda A, et al. Multiple sclerosis relapses: a multivariable analysis of residual disability determinants. Acta Neurol Scand 2009;119:126-30.

30. Patrikios P, Stadelmann C, Kutzelnigg A, et al. Remyelination is extensive in a subset of multiple sclerosis patients. Brain 2006;129(Pt 12):3165-72.

31. Damasceno A, Von Glehn F, Brandão CO, et al. Prognostic indicators for long-term disability in multiple sclerosis patients. J Neurol Sci 2013;324(1-2):29-33.

32. Cree BA, Khan O, Bourdette D, et al. Clinical characteristics of African Americans vs Caucasian Americans with multiple sclerosis. Neurology 2004;63:2039-45.

33. Naismith RT, Trinkaus K, Cross AH. Phenotype and prognosis in African-Americans with multiple sclerosis: a retrospective chart review. Mult Scler 2006;12:775-81.

34. Caillier SJ, Briggs F, Cree BA, et al. Uncoupling the roles of HLA-DRB1 and HLA-DRB5 genes in multiple sclerosis. J Immunol 2008;181:5473-80.

35. Iuliano G, Napoletano R, Esposito A. Multiple sclerosis: relapses and timing of remissions. Eur Neurol 2008;59:44-8.

36. Langer-Gould A, Popat RA, Huang SM, et al. Clinical and demographic predictors of long-term disability in patients with relapsing-remitting multiple sclerosis: a systematic review. Arch Neurol 2006;63:1686-91.

37. Katrych O, Simone TM, Azad S, Mousa SA. Disease-modifying agents in the treatment of multiple sclerosis: a review of long-term outcomes. CNS Neurol Disord Drug Targets 2009;8:512-9.

38. Paty D, Kappos L, Stam Moraga M, et al. Long-term observational efficacy and safety follow-up of the PRISMS cohort. European Committee for Treatment and Research in Multiple Sclerosis, Milan, Italy, September 17-20, 2003; abstract P555.

39. IFNB Multiple Sclerosis Study Group. Interferon beta-1b in the treatment of multiple sclerosis: final outcome of the randomized controlled trial. Neurology 1995;45:1277-85.

40. Ebers GC, Traboulsee A, Li D, et al. Analysis of clinical outcomes according to original treatment groups 16 years after the pivotal IFNB-1b trial. J Neurol Neurosurg Psychiatry 2010;81:907-12.

41. Goodin DS, Jones J, Li D, et al. Establishing long-term efficacy in chronic disease: use of recursive partitioning and propensity score adjustment to estimate outcome in MS. PLoS One 2011;6:e22444.

42. Goodin DS, Traboulsee A, Knappertz V, et al. Relationship between early clinical characteristics and long term disability outcomes: 16 year cohort study (follow-up) of the pivotal interferon β-1b trial in multiple sclerosis. J Neurol Neurosurg Psychiatry 2012;83:282-7.

43. Ford C, Goodman AD, Johnson K, et al. Continuous long-term immunomodulatory therapy in relapsing multiple sclerosis: results from the 15-year analysis of the US prospective open-label study of glatiramer acetate. Mult Scler 2010;16:342-50.

44. Trojano M, Pellegrini F, Fuiani A, et al. New natural history of interferon-beta-treated relapsing multiple sclerosis. Ann Neurol 2007;61:300-6.

45. Trojano M, Russo P, Fuiani A, et al. The Italian Multiple Sclerosis Database Network (MSDN): the risk of worsening according to IFNbeta exposure in multiple sclerosis. Mult Scler 2006;12:578-85.

46. Trojano M, Pellegrini F, Paolicelli D, et al. Real-life impact of early interferon beta therapy in relapsing multiple sclerosis. Ann Neurol 2009;66:513-20.

47. Trojano M, Paolicelli D, Tortorella C, et al. Natural history of multiple sclerosis: have available therapies impacted long-term prognosis? Neurol Clin 2011;29:309-21.

48. Brown MG, Kirby S, Skedgel C, et al. How effective are disease-modifying drugs in delaying progression in relapsing-onset MS? Neurology 2007;69:1498-507.

49. Werneck LC, Lorenzoni PJ, Radünz VA, et al. Influence of treatment in multiple sclerosis disability: an open, retrospective, non-randomized long-term analysis. Arq Neuropsiquiatr 2010;68:511-21.

50. Shirani A, Zhao Y, Karim ME, et al. Association between use of interferon beta and progression of disability in patients with relapsing-remitting multiple sclerosis. JAMA 2012;308:247-56.

51. Bergamaschi R, Quaglini S, Tavazzi E, et al. Immunomodulatory therapies delay disease progression in multiple sclerosis. Mult Scler 2012; epublished May 31, 2012.

52. Tedeholm H, Lycke J, Skoog B, et al. Time to secondary progression in patients with multiple sclerosis who were treated with first generation immunomodulating drugs. Mult Scler 2012;19:765-74.

53. Tremlett H, Zhao Y, Rieckmann P, Hutchinson M. New perspectives in the natural history of multiple sclerosis. Neurology 2010;74:2004-15.

CHAPTER 4. IS PREGNANCY A "TREATMENT" FOR MS?

1. Tafuri A, Alferink J, Moller P, et al. T cell awareness of paternal alloantigens during pregnancy. Science 1995;270:630-3.

2. Vukusic S, Hutchinson M, Hours M, et al. Pregnancy and multiple sclerosis (the PRIMS study): clinical predictors of post-partum relapse. Brain 2004;127(Pt 6):1353-60.

3. Argyriou AA, Makris N. Multiple sclerosis and reproductive risks in women. Reprod Sci 2008;15:755-64.

4. Ferrero S, Pretta S, Ragni N. Multiple sclerosis: management issues during pregnancy. Eur J Obstet Gynecol Reprod Biol 2004;115:3-9.

5. Dahl J, Myhr KM, Daltveit AK, et al. Pregnancy, delivery and birth outcome in different stages of maternal multiple sclerosis. J Neurol 2008;255:623-7.

6. Hellwig K, Brune N, Haghikia A, et al. Reproductive counselling, treatment and course of pregnancy in 73 German MS patients. Acta Neurol Scand 2008;118:24-8.

7. Roullet E, Verdier-Taillefer MH, Amarenco P, et al. Pregnancy and multiple sclerosis: a longitudinal study of 125 remittent patients. J Neuro Neurosurg Psychiatry 1993;56:1062-5.

8. Ramagopalan S, Yee I, Byrnes J, et al. Term pregnancies and the clinical characteristics of multiple sclerosis: a population based study. J Neurol Neurosurg Psychiatry 2012;83:793-5.

9. Hanulíková P, Vlk R, Meluzínová E, et al. Pregnancy and multiple sclerosis – outcomes analysis 2003-2011. Ceska Gynekol 2013;78:142-8.

10. Villard-Mackintosh L, Vessey MP. Oral contraceptives and reproductive factors in multiple sclerosis incidence.Contraception 1993;47:161-8.

11. Ponsonby AL, Lucas RM, van der Mei IA, et al. Offspring number, pregnancy, and risk of a first clinical demyelinating event: the AusImmune Study. Neurology 2012;78:867-74.

12. Keyhanian K, Davoudi V, Etemadifar M, Amin M. Better prognosis of multiple sclerosis in patients who experienced a full-term pregnancy. Eur Neurol 2012;68:150-5.

13. Koch M, Uyttenboogaart M, Heersema D, et al. Parity and secondary progression in multiple sclerosis. J Neurol Neurosurg Psychiatry 2009;80:676-8.

14. D'hooghe MB, Nagels G, Uitdehaag BM. Long-term effects of childbirth in MS. J Neurol Neurosurg Psychiatry 2010;81:38-41.

15. Soldan SS, Alvarez Retuerto AI, Sicotte NL, Voskuhl RR. Immune modulation in multiple sclerosis patients treated with the pregnancy hormone estriol. J Immunol 2003;171:6267-74.

16. Robinson DP, Klein SL. Pregnancy and pregnancy-associated hormones alter immune responses and disease pathogenesis. Horm Behav 2012;62:263-71.

17. Hughes GC. Progesterone and autoimmune disease. Autoimmun Rev 2012;11:A502-14.

18. Aristimuno C, Teijeiro R, Valor L, et al. Sex-hormone receptors pattern on regulatory T-cells: clinical implications for multiple sclerosis. Clin Exp Med 2012;12:247-55.

19. Hussain R, El-Etr M, Gaci O, et al. Progesterone and Nestorone facilitate axon remyelination: a role for progesterone receptors. Endocrinology 2011;152:3820-31.

20. Kim S, Liva SM, Dalal MA, et al. Estriol ameliorates autoimmune demyelinating disease: implications for multiple sclerosis. Neurology 1999;52:1230-8.

21. Liu H-B, Loo KK, Palaszynski K, Ashouri J, Lubahn DB, Voskuhl RR. Estrogen receptor alpha mediates estrogen's immune protection in autoimmune disease. J. Immunol 2003;171:6936-40.

22. Robinson DP, Klein SL. Pregnancy and pregnancy-associated hormones alter immune responses and disease pathogenesis. Horm Behav 2012;62:263-71.

23. Phiel KL, Henderson RA, Adelman SJ, Elloso MM. Differential estrogen receptor gene expression in human peripheral blood mononuclear cell populations. Immunol Lett 2005;97:107-13.

24. Bouman A, Heineman MJ, Faas MM. Sex hormones and the immune response in humans. Hum Reprod Update 2005;11:411-23

25. Straub RH. The complex role of estrogens in inflammation. Endocr Rev 2007;28:521-74.

26. Foroughipour A, Norbakhsh V, Najafabadi SH, Meamar R. Evaluating sex hormone levels in reproductive age women with multiple sclerosis and their relationship with disease severity. J Res Med Sci 2012;17:882-5.

27. Vukusic S, Ionescu I, El-Etr M, et al. The Prevention of Post-Partum Relapses with Progestin and Estradiol in Multiple Sclerosis (POPART'MUS) trial: rationale, objectives and state of advancement. J Neurol Sci 2009;286:114-8.

28. Vukusic S, El-Etr I, Ionescu MF, et al. The POPARTMUS French-Italian multicentric trial of Post Partum Progestin and Estriol in Multiple Sclerosis: final results. Presented at the 28th Congress of the European Committee for Treatment and Research in Multiple Sclerosis (ECTRIMS), Lyon, France, October 12, 2012; abstract 143.

29. Thorogood M, Hannaford PC. The influence of oral contraceptives on the risk of multiple sclerosis. Br J Obstet Gynaecol 1998;105:1296-9.

30. Hernan MA, Hohol MJ, Olek MJ, et al. Oral contraceptives and the incidence of multiple sclerosis. Neurology 2000;55:848-54.

31. Michel L, Foucher Y, Vukusic S, et al. Increased risk of multiple sclerosis relapse after in vitro fertilisation. J Neurol Neurosurg Psychiatry 2012;83:796-802.

32. Correale J, Farez M, Ysrraelit M. Increase in multiple sclerosis activity after assisted reproduction technology. Ann Neurol 2012;72:682-94.

33. Gilli F, Lindberg RL, Valentino P, et al. Learning from nature: pregnancy changes the expression of inflammation-related genes in patients with multiple sclerosis. PLoS One 2010;5:e8962.

34. Garcia-Segura LM, Azcoitia I, DonCarlos LL. Neuroprotection by estradiol. Prog Neurobiol 2001;63:29-60.

35. Behl C, Widmann M, Trapp T, Holsboer F. 17-beta estradiol protects neurons from oxidative stress-induced cell death in vitro. Biochem Biophys Res Commun 1995;216:473-82.

36. Goodman Y, Bruce AJ, Cheng B, Mattson MP. Estrogens attenuate and corticosterone exacerbates excitotoxicity, oxidative injury, and amyloid beta-peptide toxicity in hippocampal neurons. J Neurochem 1996;66:1836-44.

37. Harms C, Lautenschlager M, Bergk A, et al. Differential mechanisms of neuroprotection by 17 beta-estradiol in apoptotic versus necrotic neurodegeneration. J Neurosci 2001;21:2600-9.

38. Yates MA, Li Y, Chlebeck P, et al. Progesterone treatment reduces disease severity and increases IL-10 in experimental autoimmune encephalomyelitis. J Neuroimmunol 2010;220:136-9.

39. Garay L, Deniselle MC, Meyer M, et al. Protective effects of progesterone administration on axonal pathology in mice with experimental autoimmune encephalomyelitis. Brain Res 2009;1283:177-85.

40. Sicotte NL, Liva SM, Klutch R, et al. Treatment of multiple sclerosis with the pregnancy hormone estriol. Ann Neurol 2002;52:421-8.

41. Head KA. Estriol: safety and efficacy. Altern Med Rev 1998;3:101-13.

42. Taylor M. Unconventional estrogens: estriol, biest, and triest. Clin Obstet Gynecol 2001;44:864-79.

43. Cardozo L, Rekers H, Tapp A, et al. Oestriol in the treatment of postmenopausal urgency: a multicentre study. Maturitas 1993;18:47-53.

44. Hayashi T, Ito I, Kano H, et al. Estriol (E3) replacement improves endothelial function and bone mineral density in very elderly women. J Gerontol A Biol Sci Med Sci 2000;55:B183-B190.

45. Itoi H, Minakami H, Iwasaki R, Sato I. Comparison of the long-term effects of oral estriol with the effects of conjugated estrogen on serum lipid profile in early menopausal women. Maturitas 2000;36:217-22.

46. Lauritzen C. Results of a 5 years prospective study of estriol succinate treatment in patients with climacteric complaints. Hormone and Metabolic Research 1987;19:579-84.

47. Bernstein L, Ross RK, Pike MC, et al. Hormone levels in older women: a study of post-menopausal breast cancer patients and healthy population controls. Br J Cancer 1990;61:298-302.

48. Eliassen AH, Spiegelman D, Xu X, et al. Urinary estrogens and estrogen metabolites and subsequent risk of breast cancer among premenopausal women. Cancer Res 2012;72:696-706.

49. Lippman M, Monaco ME, Bolan G. Effects of estrone, estradiol, and estriol on hormone-responsive human breast cancer in long-term tissue culture. Cancer Res 1977;37:1901-7.

50. Celius E, Harbo H, Egeland T, et al. Sex and age at diagnosis are correlated with the HLA-DR2, DQ6 haplotype in multiple sclerosis. J Neurol Sci 2000;178:132-5.

51. Smith-Bouvier D, Divekar A, Sasidhar M, et al. A role for sex chromosome complement in the female bias in autoimmune disease. J Exp Med 2008;205:1099-108.

52. Spach K, Blake M, Bunn J, et al. Cutting edge: the Y chromosome controls the age-dependent experimental allergic encephalomyelitis sexual dimorphism in SJL/J mice. J Immunol 2009;182:1789-93.

53. Spach K, Hayes C. Vitamin D3 confers protection from autoimmune encephalomyelitis only in female mice. J Immunol 2005;175:4119-26.

54. Correale J, Villa A. Role of CD8+ CD25+ Foxp3+ regulatory T cells in multiple sclerosis. Ann Neurol 2010;67:625-38.

55. Tremlett H, Paty D, Devonshire V. Disability progression in multiple sclerosis is slower than previously reported. Neurology 2006;66:172-7.

56. MacKenzie-Graham A, Rinek G, Avedisian A, et al. Estrogen treatment prevents gray matter atrophy in experimental autoimmune encephalomyelitis. J Neurosci Res 2012;90:1310-23.

57. Bebo BF, Fyfe-Johnson A, Adlard K, et al. Low-dose estrogen therapy ameliorates experimental autoimmune encephalomyelitis in two different inbred mouse strains. J Immunol 2001; 166:2080-9.

58. Bebo BF, Zelinka-Vincent E, Adamus G, et al. Gonadal hormones influence the immune response to PLP 139–151 and the clinical course of relapsing experimental autoimmune encephalomyelitis. J Neuroimmunol 1998;84:122-30.

59. Pakpoor J, Goldacre R, SchmiererK, et al. Testicular hypofunction and multiple sclerosis risk: a record-linkage study. Presented at the joint Americas and European Committee for Treatment and Research in Multiple Sclerosis (ACTRIMS-ECTRIMS) meeting, Boston, MA, September 10-13, 2014; abstract LBP1.

60. Sicotte NL, Giesser BS, Tandon V, et al. Testosterone treatment in multiple sclerosis: a pilot study. Arch Neurol 2007;64:683-8.

61. Gold SM, Chalifoux S, Giesser BS, Voskuhl RR. Immune modulation and increased neurotrophic factor production in multiple sclerosis patients treated with testosterone. J Neuroinflammation 2008;5:32.

62. Langer-Gould A, Huang SM, Gupta R, et al. Exclusive breastfeeding and the risk of postpartum relapses in women with multiple sclerosis. Arch Neurol 2009;66:958-63.

63. Portaccio E, Ghezzi A, Hakiki B, et al. Breastfeeding is not related to postpartum relapses in multiple sclerosis. Neurology 2011;77:145-50.

64. Nelson LM, Franklin GM, Jones MC. Risk of multiple sclerosis exacerbation during pregnancy and breast-feeding. JAMA 1988;259:3441-3.

CHAPTER 5. WHAT ARE THE INTERFERONS?

1. Isaacs A, Lindenmann J. Virus interference. I. The interferon. Proc R Soc Lond B Biol Sci 1957;147:258-67.

2. Degré M, Dahl H, Vandvik B. Interferon in the serum and cerebrospinal fluid in patients with multiple sclerosis and other neurological disorders. Acta Neurol Scand 1976;53:152-60.

3. Neighbour PA, Bloom BR. Absence of virus-induced lymphocyte suppression and interferon production in multiple sclerosis. Proc Natl Acad Sci U S A 1979;76:476-80.

4. Jacobs L, O'Malley J, Freeman A, Ekes R. Intrathecal interferon reduces exacerbations of multiple sclerosis. Science 1981;214:1026-8.

5. Jacobs L, O'Malley JA, Freeman A, et al. Intrathecal interferon in the treatment of multiple sclerosis. Patient follow-up. Arch Neurol 1985;42:841-7.

6. Knobler RL, Panitch HS, Braheny SL, et al. Systemic alpha-interferon therapy of multiple sclerosis. Neurology 1984;34:1273-9.

7. Camenga DL, Johnson KP, Alter M, et al. Systemic recombinant alpha-2 interferon therapy in relapsing multiple sclerosis. Arch Neurol 1986;43:1239-46.

8. AUSTIMS Research Group. Interferon-alpha and transfer factor in the treatment of multiple sclerosis: a double-blind, placebo-controlled trial. J Neurol Neurosurg Psychiatry 1989;52:566-74.

9. Panitch HS, Hirsch RL, Haley AS, Johnson KP. Exacerbations of multiple sclerosis in patients treated with gamma interferon. Lancet 1987;1:893-5.

10. Panitch HS. Systemic alpha-interferon in multiple sclerosis. Long-term patient follow-up. Arch Neurol 1987;44:61-3.

11. Brod SA, Kerman RH, Nelson LD, et al. Ingested IFN-alpha has biological effects in humans with relapsing-remitting multiple sclerosis. Mult Scler 1997;3:1-7.

12. Polman C, Barkhof F, Kappos L, et al. Oral interferon beta-1a in relapsing-remitting multiple sclerosis: a double-blind randomized study. Mult Scler 2003;9:342-8.

13. The IFNB Multiple Sclerosis Study Group. Interferon beta-1b is effective in relapsing-remitting multiple sclerosis. I. Clinical results of a multicenter, randomized, double-blind, placebo-controlled trial. Neurology 1993;43:655-61.

14. The IFNB Multiple Sclerosis Study Group and the University of British Columbia MS/MRI Analysis Group. Neurology 1995;45:1277-85.

15. The Once Weekly Interferon for MS Study Group. Evidence of interferon beta-1a dose response in relapsing-remitting MS: the OWIMS Study. Neurology 1999;53:679-86.

16. Durelli L. Dose and frequency of interferon treatment matter--INCOMIN and OPTIMS. J Neurol 2003;250 Suppl 4:IV9-IV14.

17. Jacobs LD, Cookfair DL, Rudick RA, et al. Intramuscular interferon beta-1a for disease progression in relapsing multiple sclerosis. Ann Neurol 1996;39:285-94.

18. Rudick R, Goodkin D, Jacocs L, et al. Impact of interferon beta-la on in relapsing multiple sclerosis. Neurology 1997:49:358-63.

19. O'Connor PW. Key issues in the diagnosis and treatment of multiple sclerosis: an overview. Neurology 2002;59(suppl 3):1-33.

20. Rask C, Unger E, Walton M. Comparative study of Rebif to Avonex and orphan exclusivity. Food and Drug Administration memorandum, March 7, 2002.

21. PRISMS (Prevention of Relapses and Disability by Interferon b-1a Subcutaneously in Multiple Sclerosis) Study Group. Randomised double-blind placebo-controlled study of interferon b-1a in relapsing/remitting multiple sclerosis. Lancet 1998;352:1498-504.

22. Panitch H, Goodin DS, Francis G, et al. Randomized, comparative study of interferon beta-1a treatment regimens in MS: The EVIDENCE Trial. Neurology 2002;59:1496-506.

23. Schwid SR, Panitch HS. Full results of the Evidence of Interferon Dose-Response-European North American Comparative Efficacy (EVIDENCE) study: a multicenter, randomized, assessor-blinded comparison of low-dose weekly versus high-dose, high-frequency interferon beta-1a for relapsing multiple sclerosis. Clin Ther 2007;29:2031-48.

24. Jacobs LD, Beck RW, Simon JH, et al. Intramuscular interferon beta-1a therapy initiated during a first demyelinating event in multiple sclerosis. N Engl J Med 2000;343:898-904.

25. Kappos L, Polman CH, Freedman MS, et al. Treatment with interferon beta-1b delays conversion to clinically definite and McDonald MS in patients with clinically isolated syndromes. Neurology 2006;67:1242-9.

26. Comi G, De Stefano N, Freedman MS, et al. Comparison of two dosing frequencies of subcutaneous interferon beta-1a in patients with a first clinical demyelinating event suggestive of multiple sclerosis (REFLEX): a phase 3 randomised controlled trial. Lancet Neurol 2012;11:33-41.

27. European Study Group on interferon beta-1b in secondary progressive MS. Placebo-controlled multicentre randomised trial of interferon beta-1b in treatment of secondary progressive multiple sclerosis. Lancet 1998;352:1491-7.

28. Kappos L, Polman C, Pozzilli C, et al. Final analysis of the European multicenter trial on IFNbeta-1b in secondary-progressive MS. Neurology 2001;57:1969-75.

29. Secondary Progressive Efficacy Clinical Trial of Recombinant Interferon-Beta-1a in MS (SPECTRIMS) Study Group. Randomized controlled trial of interferon-beta-1a in secondary progressive MS: Clinical results. Neurology 2001;56:1496-504.

30. Li DK, Zhao GJ, Paty DW et al. Randomized controlled trial of interferon-beta-1a in secondary progressive MS: MRI results. Neurology 2001;56:1505-13.

31. Cohen JA, Cutter GR, Fischer JS, et al. Benefit of interferon beta-1a on MSFC progression in secondary progressive MS. Neurology 2002;59:679-87.

32. La Mantia L, Vacchi L, Di Pietrantonj C, et al. Interferon beta for secondary progressive multiple sclerosis. Cochrane Database Syst Rev 2012 Jan 18;1:CD005181.

33. Montalban X, Sastre-Garriga J, Tintoré M, et al. A single-center, randomized, double-blind, placebo-controlled study of interferon beta-1b on primary progressive and transitional multiple sclerosis. Mult Scler 2009;15:1195-205.

34. Rojas JI, Romano M, Ciapponi A, et al. Interferon Beta for primary progressive multiple sclerosis. Cochrane Database Syst Rev 2010 Jan 20;(1):CD006643.

35. Durelli L, Verdun E, Barbero P, et al. Every-other-day interferon beta-1b versus once-weekly interferon beta-1a for multiple sclerosis: results of a 2-year prospective randomised multicentre study (INCOMIN). Lancet 2002;359:1453-60.

36. Etemadifar M, Janghorbani M, Shaygannejad V. Comparison of Betaferon, Avonex, and Rebif in treatment of relapsing-remitting multiple sclerosis. Acta Neurol Scand 2006;113:283-7.

37. The Once Weekly Interferon for MS Study Group. Evidence of interferon beta-1a dose response in relapsing-remitting MS: the OWIMS Study. Neurology 1999;53:679-86.

38. Freedman MS, Francis GS, Sanders EA, et al. Randomized study of once-weekly interferon beta-1la therapy in relapsing multiple sclerosis: three-year data from the OWIMS study. Mult Scler 2005;11:41-5.

39. Clanet M, Radue EW, Kappos L, et al. A randomized, double-blind, dose-comparison study of weekly interferon beta-1a in relapsing MS. Neurology 2002;59:1507-17.

40. Clanet M, Kappos L, Hartung HP, et al. Interferon beta-1a in relapsing multiple sclerosis: four-year extension of the European IFNbeta-1a Dose-Comparison Study. Mult Scler 2004;10:139-44.

41. Durelli L, Barbero P, Bergui M, et al. The OPTimization of interferon for MS study: 375 microg interferon beta-1b in suboptimal responders. J Neurol 2008;255:1315-23.

42. Hurwitz BJ, Jeffery D, Arnason B, et al. Tolerability and safety profile of 12- to 28-week treatment with interferon beta-1b 250 and 500 microg QOD in patients with relapsing-remitting multiple sclerosis: a multicenter, randomized, double-blind, parallel-group pilot study. Clin Ther 2008;30:1102-12.

43. Mikol DD, Barkhof F, Chang P, et al. Comparison of subcutaneous interferon beta-1a with glatiramer acetate in patients with relapsing multiple sclerosis (the REbif vs Glatiramer Acetate in Relapsing MS Disease [REGARD] study): a multicentre, randomised, parallel, open-label trial. Lancet Neurol 2008;7:903-14.

44. Cadavid D, Wolansky LJ, Skurnick J, et al. Efficacy of treatment of MS with IFNbeta-1b or glatiramer acetate by monthly brain MRI in the BECOME study. Neurology 2009;72:1976-83.

45. O'Connor P, Filippi M, Arnason B, et al. 250 microg or 500 microg interferon beta-1b versus 20 mg glatiramer acetate in relapsing-remitting multiple sclerosis: a prospective, randomised, multicentre study. Lancet Neurol 2009;8:889-97.

46. Voskuhl RR, Gold SM. Sex-related factors in multiple sclerosis susceptibility and progression. Nat Rev Neurol 2012;8:255-63.

47. Trojano M, Pellegrini F, Paolicelli D, et al. Post-marketing of disease modifying drugs in multiple sclerosis: an exploratory analysis of gender effect in interferon beta treatment. J Neurol Sci 2009;286:109-13.

48. Rudick RA, Kappos L, Kinkel R, et al. Gender effects on intramuscular interferon beta-1a in relapsing-remitting multiple sclerosis: analysis of 1406 patients. Mult Scler 2011;17:353-60.

49. Contasta I, Totaro R, Pellegrini P, et al. A gender-related action of IFNbeta-therapy was found in multiple sclerosis. J Transl Med 2012;10:223.

50. Moldovan IR, Cotleur AC, Zamor N, et al. Multiple sclerosis patients show sexual dimorphism in cytokine responses to myelin antigens. J Neuroimmunol 2008;193:161-9.

51. Enevold C, Oturai AB, Sørensen PS, et al. Polymorphisms of innate pattern recognition receptors, response to interferon-beta and development of neutralizing antibodies in multiple sclerosis patients. Mult Scler 2010;16:942-9.

52. Gold R, Kappos L, Arnold DL, et al. Placebo-controlled phase 3 study of oral BG-12 for relapsing multiple sclerosis. N Engl J Med 2012;367:1098-107.

53. Kister I, Chamot E, Bacon JH, et al. Rapid disease course in African Americans with multiple sclerosis. Neurology 2010;75:217-23.

54. Cree BA, Al-Sabbagh A, Bennett R, Goodin D. Response to interferon beta-1a treatment in African American multiple sclerosis patients. Arch Neurol 2005;62:1681-3.

55. Klineova S, Nicholas J, Walker A. Response to disease modifying therapies in African Americans with multiple sclerosis. Ethn Dis 2012;22:221-5.

56. Gupta S, Varadarajulu R, Ganjoo RK. Beta-interferons in multiple sclerosis: a single center experience in India. Klineova S, Nicholas J, Walker A Ann Indian Acad Neurol 2010;13:132-5.

57. Chan KH, Tsang KL, Ho PW, et al. Clinical outcome of relapsing remitting multiple sclerosis among Hong Kong Chinese. Clin Neurol Neurosurg 2011;113:617-22.

58. Logan-Clubb L, Stacy M. An open-labelled assessment of adverse effects associated with interferon 1-beta in the treatment of multiple sclerosis. J Neurosci Nurs 1995;27:344-7.

59. Rice GP, Ebers GC, Lublin FD, Knobler RL. Ibuprofen treatment versus gradual introduction of interferon beta-1b in patients with MS. Neurology 1999;52:1893-5.

60. Reess J, Haas J, Gabriel K, et al. Both paracetamol and ibuprofen are equally effective in managing flu-like symptoms in relapsing-remitting multiple sclerosis patients during interferon beta-1a (AVONEX) therapy. Mult Scler 2002;8:15-8.

61. Visser LH, van der Zande A. Reasons patients give to use or not to use immunomodulating agents for multiple sclerosis. Eur J Neurol 2011;18:1343-9.

62. Balak DM, Hengstman GJ, Çakmak A, Thio HB. Cutaneous adverse events associated with disease-modifying treatment in multiple sclerosis: a systematic review. Mult Scler 2012;18:1705-17.

63. Beer K, Muller M, Hew-Winzeler AM, et al. The prevalence of injection-site reactions with disease-modifying therapies and their effect on adherence in patients with multiple sclerosis: an observational study. Neurology 2011;11:144.

64. Reder AT, Ebers GC, Traboulsee A, et al. Cross-sectional study assessing long-term safety of interferon-beta-1b for relapsing-remitting MS. Neurology 2010;74:1877-85.
65. Monzani F, Caraccio N, Meucci G, et al. Effect of 1-year treatment with interferon-beta1b on thyroid function and autoimmunity in patients with multiple sclerosis. Eur J Endocrinol 1999;141:325-31.
66. Durelli L, Ferrero B, Oggero A, et al. Autoimmune events during interferon beta-1b treatment for multiple sclerosis. J Neurol Sci 1999;162:74-83.
67. Evans C, Tam J, Kingwell E, et al. Long-term persistence with the immunomodulatory drugs for multiple sclerosis: a retrospective database study. Clin Ther 2012;34:341-50.
68. Meyniel C, Spelman T, Jokubaitis VG, et al. Country, sex, EDSS change and therapy choice independently predict treatment discontinuation in multiple sclerosis and clinically isolated syndrome. PLoS One 2012;7:e38661.
69. Wong J, Gomes T, Mamdani M, et al. Adherence to multiple sclerosis disease-modifying therapies in Ontario is low. Can J Neurol Sci 2011;38:429-33.
70. Steinberg SC, Faris RJ, Chang CF, et al. Impact of adherence to interferons in the treatment of multiple sclerosis: a non-experimental, retrospective, cohort study. Clin Drug Investig 2010;30:89-100.
71. Rinon A, Buch M, Holley D, Verdun E. The MS Choices Survey: findings of a study assessing physician and patient perspectives on living with and managing multiple sclerosis. Patient Prefer Adherence 2011;5:629-43.

CHAPTER 6. WHAT IS COPAXONE?

1. Arnon R. The development of Cop 1 (Copaxone), an innovative drug for the treatment of multiple sclerosis: personal reflections. Immunol Lett 1996;50:1-15.
2. Rivers TM, Schwentker FF. Encephalomyelitis accompanied by myelin destruction experimentally produced in monkeys. J Exp Med 1935;61:689-702.
3. Paterson PY. Experimental allergic encephalomyelitis and autoimmune disease. Adv Immunol 1966;5:131-208.
4. Teitelbaum D, Meshorer A, Hirshfeld T, et al. Suppression of experimental allergic encephalomyelitis by a synthetic polypeptide. Eur J Immunol 1971;1:242-8.
5. Bornstein MB, Miller AE, Teitelbaum D, et al. Treatment of multiple sclerosis with a synthetic polypeptide: preliminary results. Trans Am Neurol Assoc 1980;105:348-50.
6. Bornstein MB, Miller AI, Teitelbaum D, et al. Multiple sclerosis: trial of a synthetic polypeptide. Ann Neurol 1982;11:317-9.
7. Bornstein MB, Miller A, Slagle S, et al. A pilot trial of Cop 1 in exacerbating-remitting multiple sclerosis. N Engl J Med 1987;317:408-14.
8. Shaw SY, Laursen RA, Lee MB. Analogous amino acid sequences in myelin proteolipid and viral proteins. FEBS Lett 1986;207:266-70.
9. Bar-Or A, Oliveira EM, Anderson DE, et al. Molecular pathogenesis of multiple sclerosis. J Neuroimmunol 1999; 100:252-9.
10. Wucherpfennig KW, Strominger JL. Molecular mimicry in T cell-mediated autoimmunity: viral peptides activate human T cell clones specific for myelin basic protein. Cell 1995;80:695-705.
11. Tejada-Simon MV, Zang YC, Hong J, et al. Cross-reactivity with myelin basic protein and human herpesvirus-6 in multiple sclerosis. Ann Neurol 2003;53:189-97.

12. Croxford JL, Olson JK, Anger HA, et al. Initiation and exacerbation of autoimmune demyelination of the central nervous system via virus-induced molecular mimicry: implications for the pathogenesis of multiple sclerosis. J Virol 2005;79:8581-90.

13. Fridkis-Hareli M, Teitelbaum D, Gurevich E, et al. Direct binding of myelin basic protein and synthetic copolymer 1 to class II major histocompatibility complex molecules on living antigen-presenting cells – specificity and promiscuity. Proc Natl Acad Sci USA 1994;91:4872-6.

14. Ben-Nun A, Mendel I, Bakimer R, et al. The autoimmune reactivity to myelin oligodendrocyte glycoprotein (MOG) in multiple sclerosis is potentially pathogenic: effect of copolymer 1 on MOG-induced disease. J Neurol 1996;243:S14-S22.

15. Teitelbaum D, Fridkis-Hareli M, Arnon R, et al. Copolymer 1 inhibits chronic relapsing experimental allergic encephalomyelitis induced by proteolipid protein (PLP) peptides in mice and interferes with PLP-specific T cell responses. J Neuroimmunol 1996;64: 209-17.

16. Aharoni R, Teitelbaum D, Sela M, et al. Copolymer 1 induces T cells of the T helper type 2 that crossreact with myelin basic protein and suppress experimental autoimmune encephalomyelitis. Proc Natl Acad Sci USA 1997;94:10821-6.

17. Chen M, Gran B, Costello K, et al. Glatiramer acetate induces a Th2-biased response and crossreactivity with myelin basic protein in patients with MS. Mult Scler 2001;7: 209-19.

18. Dhib-Jalbut S, Chen M, Said A, et al. Glatiramer acetate-reactive peripheral blood mononuclear cells respond to multiple myelin antigens with a Th2-biased phenotype. J Neuroimmunol 2003;140:163-71.

19. Johnson KP, Brooks BR, Cohen JA, et al. Copolymer 1 reduces relapse rate and improves disability in relapsing-remitting multiple sclerosis: results of a phase III multicenter, double-blind, placebo-controlled trial. Neurology 1995;45: 1268-76.

20. Liu C, Blumhardt LD. Benefits of glatiramer acetate on disability in relapsing-remitting multiple sclerosis. An analysis by area under disability/time curves. The Copolymer 1 Multiple Sclerosis Study Group. J Neurol Sci 2000;181:33-7.

21. Ge Y, Grossman RI, Udupa JK, et al. Glatiramer acetate (Copaxone) treatment in relapsing-remitting MS: quantitative MR assessment. Neurology 2000;54:813-7.

22. Comi G, Filippi M, Wolinsky JS. European/Canadian multicenter, double-blind, randomized, placebo-controlled study of the effects of glatiramer acetate on magnetic resonance imaging--measured disease activity and burden in patients with relapsing multiple sclerosis. European/Canadian Glatiramer Acetate Study Group. Ann Neurol 2001;49:290-7.

23. Wolinsky JS, Narayana PA, Johnson KP, et al. United States open-label glatiramer acetate extension trial for relapsing multiple sclerosis: MRI and clinical correlates. Multiple Sclerosis Study Group and the MRI Analysis Center. Mult Scler 2001;7:33-41.

24. O'Connor P, Canadian Multiple Sclerosis Working Group. Key issues in the diagnosis and treatment of multiple sclerosis. An overview. Neurology 2002;59(6 Suppl 3):S1-33.

25. Johnson KP, Brooks BR, Cohen JA, et al. Extended use of glatiramer acetate (Copaxone) is well tolerated and maintains its clinical effect on multiple sclerosis relapse rate and degree of disability. Copolymer 1 Multiple Sclerosis Study Group. Neurology 1998;50:701-8.

26. Johnson KP, Brooks BR, Ford CC, et al. Sustained clinical benefits of glatiramer acetate in relapsing multiple sclerosis patients observed for 6 years. Copolymer 1 Multiple Sclerosis Study Group. Mult Scler 2000;6:255-66.

27. Johnson KP, Ford CC, Lisak RP, et al. Neurologic consequence of delaying glatiramer acetate therapy for multiple sclerosis: 8-year data. Acta Neurol Scand 2005;111:42-7.

28. Ford CC, Johnson KP, Lisak RP, et al. A prospective open-label study of glatiramer acetate: Over a decade of continuous use in MS patients. Mult Scler 2006;12:309-20.

29. Ford C, Goodman AD, Johnson K, et al. Continuous long-term immunomodulatory therapy in relapsing multiple sclerosis: results from the 15-year analysis of the US prospective open-label study of glatiramer acetate. Mult Scler 2010;16:342-50.

30. Ford C, Ladkani D, on behalf of the US Open-label Glatiramer Acetate Study Group. Twenty years of continuous treatment of multiple sclerosis with glatiramer acetate 20 mg daily: long-term clinical results of the US open-label extension study. Presented at the 29th Congress of the European Committee for Treatment and Research in Multiple Sclerosis, Copenhagen, Denmark, October 2-5, 2013; abstract P577.

31. Polman CH, Reingold SC, Banwell B, et al. Diagnostic criteria for multiple sclerosis: 2010 revisions to the McDonald criteria. Ann Neurol 2011;69:292-302.

32. Jacobs LD. Beck RW, Simon JH, et al. Intramuscular interferon beta-1a therapy initiated during a first demyelinating event in multiple sclerosis. N Engl J Med 2000; 343:898-904.

33. Comi G, Martinelli V, Rodegher M, et al. Effect of glatiramer acetate on conversion to clinically definite multiple sclerosis in patients with clinically isolated syndrome (PreCISe study): a randomised, double-blind, placebo-controlled trial. Lancet 2009;374:1503-11.

34. Wolinsky JS, Narayana PA, O'Connor P, et al. Glatiramer acetate in primary progressive multiple sclerosis: results of a multinational, multicenter, double-blind, placebo-controlled trial. Ann Neurol 2007;61:14-24.

35. Faria AM, Weiner HL. Oral tolerance. Immunol Rev 2005;206:232-59.

36. Weiner HL, Mackin GA, Matsui M, et al. Double-blind pilot trial of oral tolerization with myelin antigens in multiple sclerosis. Science 1993;259:1321-4.

37. Aharoni R, Meshorer A, Sela M, et al. Oral treatment of mice with copolymer 1 (glatiramer acetate) results in the accumulation of specific Th2 cells in the central nervous system. J Neuroimmunol 2002;126:58-68.

38. Filippi M, Wolinsky JS, Comi G, et al. Effects of oral glatiramer acetate on clinical and MRI-monitored disease activity in patients with relapsing multiple sclerosis: a multicentre, double-blind, randomised, placebo-controlled study. Lancet Neurol 2006;5:213-20.

39. Cohen JA, Rovaris M, Goodman AD, et al. Randomized, double-blind, dose-comparison study of glatiramer acetate in relapsing-remitting MS. Neurology 2007;68:939-44.

40. Comi G, Cohen JA, Arnold DL, et al. Phase III dose-comparison study of glatiramer acetate for multiple sclerosis. Ann Neurol 2011;69:75-82.

41. Flechter S, Kott E, Steiner-Birmanns B, et al. Copolymer 1 (glatiramer acetate) in relapsing forms of multiple sclerosis: open multicenter study of alternate-day administration. Clin Neuropharmacol 2002;25:11-5.

42. Caon C, Perumal J, Tselis A, et al. Twice-weekly versus daily glatiramer acetate: results of a randomized, rater-blinded prospective clinical trial clinical and MRI study in relapsing-remitting MS. Presented at the American Academy of Neurology annual meeting, Toronto, ON, April 11-15, 2010; abstract S11.002.

43. Khan O, Rieckmann P, Boyko A, et al. A multinational, multicenter, randomized, placebo-controlled, double-blind study to assess the efficacy, safety, and tolerability of glatiramer acetate 40 mg injection three times a week in subjects with RRMS: efficacy and safety results of the GALA Study. Abstract S01.005. Presented at the American Academy of Neurology annual meeting, San Diego CA, March 16- 23, 2013.

44. EP Vantage. Gala could lengthen Copaxone's life but litigation and competitors threaten. June 15, 2012. www.epvantage.com/ Universal/ View.aspx?type= Story&id=301783&isEPVantage=yes.

45. Kipnis J, Schwartz M. Dual action of glatiramer acetate (Cop-1) in the treatment of CNS autoimmune and neurodegenerative disorders. Trends Mol Med 2002;8:319-23.

46. Drago F, Brusati C, Mancardi G, et al. Localized lipoatrophy after glatiramer acetate injection in patients with remitting-relapsing multiple sclerosis. Arch Dermatol 1999;135:1277-8.

47. Edgar CM, Brunet DG, Fenton P, et al. Lipoatrophy in patients with multiple sclerosis on glatiramer acetate. Can J Neurol Sci 2004;31:58-63.

48. Mancardi GL. Localized lipoatrophy after prolonged treatment with copolymer-1. J Neurol 2000;247:220-1.

49. Lebrun C, Bertagna M, Cohen M. Cutaneous side-effects of immunomodulators in MS. Int MS J 2011;17:88-94.

50. Hashimoto S, Ball NJ, Tremlett H. Progressive lipoatrophy after cessation of glatiramer acetate injections: a case report. Mult Scler 2009;15:521-2.

CHAPTER 7. WHAT IS TYSABRI?

1. Pischel KD, Bluestein HG, Woods VL Jr. Very late activation antigens (VLA) are human leukocyte-neuronal crossreactive cell surface antigens. J Exp Med 1986;164:393-406.

2. Yednock TA, Cannon C, Fritz LC, et al. Prevention of experimental autoimmune encephalomyelitis by antibodies against alpha 4 beta 1 integrin. Nature 1992;356:63-6.

3. Sheremata WA, Vollmer TL, Stone LA, et al. A safety and pharmacokinetic study of intravenous natalizumab in patients with MS. Neurology 1999;52:1072-4.

4. Tubridy N, Behan PO, Capildeo R, et al. The effect of anti-alpha4 integrin antibody on brain lesion activity in MS. The UK Antegren Study Group. Neurology 1999;53:466-72.

5. Miller DH, Khan OA, Sheremata WA, et al. A controlled trial of natalizumab for relapsing multiple sclerosis. N Engl J Med 2003;348:15-23.

6. Bryan WW, et al. Center for Drug Research and Evaluation. Medical Review, application 125104. Parts 1-IV. November 23, 2004.

7. Tysabri (natalizumab) Product Monograph. Biogen Idec., 2004.

8. Astrom KE, Mancall EL, Richardson EP Jr. Progressive multifocal leuko-encephalopathy; a hitherto unrecognized complication of chronic lymphatic leukaemia and Hodgkin's disease. Brain 1958;81:93-111.

9. Brooks BR, Walker DL. Progressive multifocal leukoencephalopathy. Neurol Clin 1984;2:299-313.

10. Padgett BL, Walker DL, ZuRhein GM, et al. Cultivation of papova-like virus from human brain with progressive multifocal leucoencephalopathy. Lancet 1971;1:1257-60.

11. Miller JR, Barrett RE, Britton CB, et al. Progressive multifocal leukoencephalopathy in a male homosexual with T-cell immune deficiency. N Engl J Med 1982;307:1436-8.

12. Selik RM, Karon JM, Ward JW. Effect of the human immunodeficiency virus epidemic on mortality from opportunistic infections in the United States in 1993. J Infect Dis 1997;176:632-6.

13. Padgett BL, Walker DL. Prevalence of antibodies in human sera against JC virus, an isolate from a case of progressive multifocal leukoencephalopathy. J Infect Dis 1973;127:467-70.

14. Bofill-Mas S, Girones R. Excretion and transmission of JCV in human populations. J Neurovirol 2001; 7:345-9.

15. Monaco MC, Jensen PN, Hou J, et al. Detection of JC virus DNA in human tonsil tissue: evidence for site of initial viral infection. J Virol 1998;72:9918-23.

16. Dorries K, ter Meulen V. Progressive multifocal leucoencephalopathy: detection of papovavirus JC in kidney tissue. J Med Virol 1983;11:307-17.

17. Diotti RA, Nakanishi A, Clementi N, et al. JC Polyomavirus (JCV) and Monoclonal Antibodies: Friends or Potential Foes? Clin Dev Immunol 2013;2013:967581.

18. Maginnis MS, Atwood WJ. JCV: An oncogenic virus in animals and humans? Semin Cancer Biol 2009;19:261-9.

19. Khalil K, White MK. Human demyelinating disease and the polyomavirus JCV. Mult Scler 2006;12:133-42.

20. Kleinschmidt-DeMasters BK, Tyler KL. Progressive multifocal leukoencephalopathy complicating treatment with natalizumab and interferon beta-1a for multiple sclerosis. N Engl J Med 2005;353:369-74.

21. Langer-Gould A, Atlas SW, Green AJ, et al. Progressive multifocal leukoencephalopathy in a patient treated with natalizumab. N Engl J Med 2005;353: 375-81.

22. Van Assche G, Van Ranst M, Sciot R, et al. Progressive multifocal leukoencephalopathy after natalizumab therapy for Crohn's disease. N Engl J Med 2005; 353:362-8.

23. Berger T, Deisenhammer F. Progressive multifocal leukoencephalopathy, natalizumab, and multiple sclerosis. N Engl J Med 2005;353:1744-6.

24. Alvarez-Cermeno JC, Masjuan J, Villar LM, et al. Progressive multifocal leukoencephalopathy, natalizumab, and multiple sclerosis. N Engl J Med 2005;353: 1744-6.

25. Langer-Gould A, Atlas SW, Pelletier D. Progressive multifocal leukoencephalopathy, natalizumab, and multiple sclerosis. N Engl J Med 2005; 353:1744-6.

26. Clanet M. Therapeutic developments in MS: Report from the 57th Annual Meeting of the American Academy of Neurology (AAN), 9-16 April 2005, Miami Beach, Florida, USA. Int MS J 2005;12:69-70.

27. Yousry TA, Major EO, Ryschkewitsch C, et al. Evaluation of patients treated with natalizumab for progressive multifocal leukoencephalopathy. N Engl J Med 2006;354: 924-33.

28. Bloomgren G, Richman S, Hotermans C, et al. Updated incidence of progressive multifocal leukoencephalopathy in natalizumab-treated multiple sclerosis patients stratified by established risk factors. Neurology 2012;78(suppl 1):S41.001.

29. Biogen Idec Medical Information Sheet. Tysabri (natalizumab) safety update, 17 August 2012. www.tapp.com.au/members/Tysabri_Safety_Update_160812.pdf. Accessed August 1, 2013.

30. http://chefarztfrau.de/?page_id=716. Accessed July 12, 2014.

31. http://chefarztfrau.de/?page_id=716. Accessed January 9, 2015.

32. Tysabri (natalizumab) Product Monograph. Biogen Idec, revised 12/2013.

33. Polman CH, O'Connor PW, Havrdova E, et al. Randomized, placebo-controlled trial of natalizumab for relapsing multiple sclerosis. N Engl J Med 2006;354:899-910.

34. Rudick RA, Stuart WH, Calabresi PA, et al. Natalizumab plus interferon beta-1a for relapsing multiple sclerosis. N Engl J Med 2006;354:911-23.

35. Goodin DS, Cohen BA, O'Connor P, et al. Assessment: The use of natalizumab (Tysabri) for the treatment of multiple sclerosis (an evidence-based review) : Report of the Therapeutics and Technology Assessment Subcommittee of the American Academy of Neurology. Neurology 2008;71;766-73.

36. Goodman AD, Rossman H, Bar-Or A, et al. GLANCE: Results of a phase 2, randomized, double-blind, placebo-controlled study. Neurology 2009;72:806-12.

37. Prosperini L, Gianni C, Leonardi L, et al. Escalation to natalizumab or switching among immunomodulators in relapsing multiple sclerosis. Mult Scler 2012;18:64-71.

38. Lee P, Plavina T, Castro A, et al. A second-generation ELISA (STRATIFY JCV™ DxSelect™) for detection of JC virus antibodies in human serum and plasma to support progressive multifocal leukoencephalopathy risk stratification. J Clin Virol 2013;57:141-6.

39. Bettin M, Lin J, Sadiq S. Accurate risk assessment for the development of PML in natalizumab treated MS patients requires CSF analysis. Neurology 2012;78(suppl 1):P07.056.

40. Chan A, Trampe A-K, Hemmelmann C, et al. Anti-JC virus antibodies in a large German natalizumab-treated multiple sclerosis cohort. Neurology 2012;78(suppl 1):P02.137.

41. Berger JR, Houff SA, Gurwell J, et al. JC virus antibody status underestimates infection rates. Ann Neurol 2013;74:84-90.

42. Plavina T, Lee S, Berman M, et al. Longitudinal stability of anti-JC virus antibody status in multiple sclerosis patients: results of STRATIFY-1. American Academy of Neurology annual meeting, San Diego CA, March 16-23, 2013; abstract S30.001.

43. Lanzillo R, Liuzzi R, Amato L, et al. JC virus antibodies index on natalizumab treatment: fluctuations and seroconversion. Presented at the 29th Congress of the European Committee for Treatment and Research in Multiple Sclerosis, Copenhagen, Denmark, October 2-5, 2013; abstract P599.

44. Houff SA, Berger JR. The bone marrow, B cells, and JC virus. J Neurovirol 2008;14:341-3.

45. Lindberg RL, Achtnichts L, Hoffmann F, et al. Natalizumab alters transcriptional expression profiles of blood cell subpopulations of multiple sclerosis patients. J Neuroimmunol 2008;194:153-64.

46. Yao K, Gagnon S, Akhyani N, et al. Reactivation of human herpesvirus-6 in natalizumab treated multiple sclerosis patients. PLoS ONE 2008; 3:2028.

47. Lanzillo R, Liuzzi R, Vallefuoco L, et al. Anti-JC virus antibodies index and JCV DNA concordance and markers of active viral replication: true exposure to JCV virus in natalizumab treated patients. Presented at the 29th Congress of the European Committee for Treatment and Research in Multiple Sclerosis, Copenhagen, Denmark, October 2-5, 2013; abstract P1067.

48. van Pesch V, Algoed L, Boucquey D, et al. Use of the JC virus stratify assay in a cohort of natalizumab-treated patients from Belgium. Comparative results between 2011 and 2012. Presented at the 29th Congress of the European Committee for Treatment and Research in Multiple Sclerosis, Copenhagen, Denmark, October 2-5, 2013; abstract P1070.

49. Williamson E, Aparicio J, Buckbinder L, et al. Update on experience with natalizumab use, JCV antibody testing & treatment decisions at the university of Southern California MS center – including sex differences. American Academy of Neurology annual meeting, San Diego CA, March 16-23, 2013; abstract P01.213.

50. Foley J. Natalizumab Related PML: An evolving risk stratification paradigm. American Academy of Neurology annual meeting, San Diego CA, March 16-23, 2013; abstract S30.002.

51. Zhovtis Ryerson L, Wiener B, Elyashiv M, et al. Alternate-month dosing schedule for natalizumab. Presented at the 29th Congress of the European Committee for Treatment and Research in Multiple Sclerosis, Copenhagen, Denmark, October 2-5, 2013; abstract P1068.

52. Tornatore C, Erwin A. Dosing natalizumab every other month following 2 years of monthly dosing. Neurology 2012;78(suppl 1):PD5.003.

53. Rudick RA, Miller D, Hass S, et al. Health-related quality of life in multiple sclerosis: effects of natalizumab. Ann Neurol 2007;62:335-46.

54. O'Connor PW, Goodman A, Kappos L, et al. Disease activity return during natalizumab treatment interruption in patients with multiple sclerosis. Neurology 2011;76:1858-65.

55. Stuve O, Cravens PD, Frohman EM, et al. Immunologic, clinical, and radiologic status 14 months after cessation of natalizumab therapy. Neurology 2009;72:396-401.

56. Schaaf SM, Pitt D, Racke MK. What happens when natalizumab therapy is stopped? Expert Rev Neurother 2011;11:1247-50.

57. Kerbrat A, Le Page E, Leray E, et al. Natalizumab and drug holiday in clinical practice: an observational study in very active relapsing remitting multiple sclerosis patients. J Neurol Sci 2011;308:98-102.

58. Sangalli F, Moiola L, Barcella V, et al. What to expect after natalizumab in every-day clinical practice. Neurology 2012;78 (suppl 1):P06.169.

59. Rossi S, Motta C, Studer V, et al. Effect of glatiramer acetate on disease reactivation in MS patients discontinuing natalizumab. Eur J Neurol 2013;20:87-94.

60. Havla J, Gerdes LA, Meinl I, et al. De-escalation from natalizumab in multiple sclerosis: recurrence of disease activity despite switching to glatiramer acetate. J Neurol 2011;258:1665-9.

61. Fox R, Cree B, De Seze J, et al. RESTORE study: effects of natalizumab interruption on multiple sclerosis disease activity (abstract DX88). Int J MS Care 2012;14(suppl 2): 4.

62. Rinaldi F, Seppi D, Calabrese M, et al. Switching therapy from natalizumab to fingolimod in relapsing-remitting multiple sclerosis: clinical and magnetic resonance imaging findings. Mult Scler 2012;18:1640-3.

63. Laroni A, Brogi D, Milesi V, et al. Early switch to fingolimod may decrease the risk of disease recurrence after natalizumab interruption. Mult Scler 2012;19:1236-7.

64. Havla J, Tackenberg B, Hellwig K, et al. Fingolimod reduces recurrence of disease activity after natalizumab withdrawal in multiple sclerosis. J Neurol 2012;260:1382-7.

65. de Seze J, Ongagna J, Zaenker C, et al. Reduction of washout delay between Tysabri and Gilenya: a regional real-life study. Presented at the 29th Congress of the European Committee for Treatment and Research in Multiple Sclerosis, Copenhagen, Denmark, October 2-5, 2013; abstract P634.

CHAPTER 8. WHAT IS GILENYA?

1. Fujita T, Inoue K, Yamamoto S, et al. Fungal metabolites. Part 11. A potent immunosuppressive activity found in *Isaria sinclairii* metabolite. J Antibiot 1994;47:208-15.

2. Adachi K, Kohara T, Nakao N, et al. Design, synthesis, and structure-activity relationships of 2-substituted-2-amino-1,3-propanediols: discovery of a novel immunosuppressant, FTY720. Bioorg Med Chem Lett 1995;5:853-6.

3. Chun J, Brinkmann V. A mechanistically novel, first oral therapy for multiple sclerosis: the development of fingolimod (FTY720, Gilenya). Discov Med 2011;12:213-28.

4. Maki T, Gottschalk R, Monaco AP. Prevention of autoimmune diabetes by FTY720 in nonobese diabetic mice. Transplantation 2002;74:1684-6.

5. Okazaki H, Hirata D, Kamimura T, et al. Effects of FTY720 in MRL-lpr/lpr mice: therapeutic potential in systemic lupus erythematosus. J Rheumatol 2002;29:707-16.

6. Chiba K, Yanagawa Y, Masubuchi Y, et al. FTY720, a novel immunosuppressant, induces sequestration of circulating mature-lymphocytes by acceleration of lymphocyte homing in rats: I. FTY720 selectively decreases the number of circulating mature lymphocytes by acceleration of lymphocyte homing. *J Immunol* 1998;160:5037-44.

7. Chun J, Hartung H-P. Mechanism of action of oral fingolimod (FTY720) in multiple sclerosis. Clin Neuropharmacol 2010;33:91-101.

8. Sinha RK, Park C, Hwang IY, et al. B lymphocytes exit lymph nodes through cortical lymphatic sinusoids by a mechanism independent of sphingosine-1-phosphate-mediated chemotaxis.Immunity 2009;30:434-46.

9. Brinkmann V, Metzler B, Matloubian M, et al. The mode of action of fingolimod (FTY720), an oral sphingosine 1-phosphate receptor modulator that is highly effective in human multiple sclerosis (phase II). Mult Scler 2006;12:S100.

10. Mehling M, Brinkmann V, Antel J, et al. FTY720 therapy exerts differential effects on T cell subsets in multiple sclerosis. Neurology 2008;71:1261-7.

11. Pinschewer DD, Ochsenbein AF, Odermatt B, et al. FTY720 Immunosuppression impairs effector T cell peripheral homing without affecting induction, expansion, and memory. J Immunol 2000;164:5761-70.

12. Francis G, Kappos L, O'Connor P, et al. Lymphocytes and fingolimod – temporal pattern and relationship with infections. Presented at the 26th Congress of the European Committee for Treatment and Research in Multiple Sclerosis (ECTRIMS), Gothenburg, Sweden, October 13-16, 2010; abstract P442.

13. Kappos L, Antel J, Comi J, et al. Oral fingolimod (FTY720) for relapsing multiple sclerosis. N Engl J Med 2006;355:1124-40.

14. O'Connor P, Comi G, Montalban X, et al. Oral fingolimod (FTY720) in multiple sclerosis: two-year results of a phase II extension study. Neurology 2009;72:73-9.

15. Kovarik JM, Schmouder R, Barilla D, et al. Single-dose FTY720 pharmacokinetics, food effect, and pharmacological responses in healthy subjects. Br J Clin Pharmacol 2004;57:586-91.

16. Tedesco-Silva H, Mourad G, Kahan BD, et al. FTY720, a novel immunomodulator: efficacy and safety results from the first phase 2A study in de novo renal transplantation. Transplantation 2005;79:1553-60.

17. Kahan BD, Karlix JL, Ferguson RM, et al. Pharmacodynamics, pharmacokinetics, and safety of multiple doses of FTY720 in stable renal transplant patients: a multicenter, randomized, placebo-controlled, phase I study. Transplantation 2003;76:1079-84.

18. Salvadori M, Budde K, Charpentier B, et al. FTY720 versus MMF with cyclosporine in de novo renal transplantation: a 1-year, randomized controlled trial in Europe and Australasia. Am J Transplant 2006;6:2912-21.

19. Kovarik JM, Schmouder R, Barilla D, et al. Multiple-dose FTY720: tolerability, pharmacokinetics, and lymphocyte responses in healthy subjects. J Clin Pharmacol 2004;44:532-7.

20. Kappos L, Radue EW, O'Connor P, et al. A placebo-controlled trial of oral fingolimod in relapsing multiple sclerosis. N Engl J Med 2010;362:387-401.

21. Cohen JA, Barkhof F, Comi G, et al. Oral fingolimod or intramuscular interferon for relapsing multiple sclerosis. N Engl J Med 2010;362:402-15.

22. Calabresi PA, Radue EW, Goodin D, et al. Safety and efficacy of fingolimod in patients with relapsing-remitting multiple sclerosis (FREEDOMS II): a double-blind, randomised, placebo-controlled, phase 3 trial. Lancet Neurol 2014;13:545-556.

23. Roskell NS, Zimovetz EA, Rycroft CE, et al. Annualized relapse rate of first-line treatments for multiple sclerosis: a meta-analysis, including indirect comparisons versus fingolimod. Curr Med Res Opin 2012;28:767-80.

24. Del Santo F, Maratea D, Fadda V, et al. Treatments for relapsing-remitting multiple sclerosis: summarising current information by network meta-analysis. Eur J Clin Pharmacol 2012;68:441-8.

25. Ontaneda D, Cohen JA. Potential mechanisms of efficacy and adverse effects in the use of fingolimod (FTY720). Expert Rev Clin Pharmacol 2011;4:567-70.

26. Vollmer T, Jeffery D, Goodin D, et al. Long-term safety of fingolimod in patients with relapsing-remitting multiple sclerosis: results from phase 3 FREEDOMS II extension study. Presented at the American Academy of Neurology annual meeting, San Diego CA, March 16- 23, 2013; abstract P01.165.

27. Schreiber RD, Old LJ, Smyth MJ. Cancer immunoediting: integrating immunity's roles in cancer suppression and promotion. Science 2011;331:1565-70.

28. Lorvik KB, Bogen B, Corthay A. Fingolimod blocks immunosurveillance of myeloma and B-cell lymphoma resulting in cancer development in mice. Blood 2012;119:2176-7.

29. Long JS, Fujiwara Y, Edwards J, et al. Sphingosine 1-phosphate receptor 4 uses HER2 (ERBB2) to regulate extracellular signal regulated kinase-1/2 in MDA-MB-453 breast cancer cells. J Biol Chem 2010;285:35957-66.

30. Zhang N, Qi Y, Wadham C, et al. FTY720 induces necrotic cell death and autophagy in ovarian cancer cells: a protective role of autophagy. Autophagy 2010;6:1157-67.

31. Pchejetski D, Bohler T, Brizuela L, et al. FTY720 (fingolimod) sensitizes prostate cancer cells to radiotherapy by inhibition of sphingosine kinase-1. Cancer Res 2010;70:8651-661.

32. Koyrakh L, Roman MI, Brinkmann V, Wickman K. The heart rate decrease caused by acute FTY720 administration is mediated by the G protein-gated potassium channel I. Am J Transplant 2005;5:529-36.

33. Schmouder R, Hariry S, David OJ. Placebo-controlled study of the effects of fingolimod on cardiac rate and rhythm and pulmonary function in healthy volunteers. Eur J Clin Pharmacol 2012;68:355-62.

34. Bermel R, Ontaneda D, Hara-Cleaver C, et al. Cardiovascular effects and safety of fingolimod in clinical practice. Neurology 2012;78(suppl 1): P04.138.

35. Kovarik JM, Lu M, Riviere GJ, et al. The effect on heart rate of combining single-dose fingolimod with steady-state atenolol or diltiazem in healthy subjects. Eur J Clin Pharmacol 2008;64:457-63.

36. DiMarco J, Collins W, Francis G, et al. Pooled analyses of the transient and long-term effects of fingolimod (FTY720) on cardiovascular parameters in phase 3 studies in patients with multiple sclerosis. Presented at the American Academy of Neurology annual meeting, Honolulu HI, April 9- 16, 2011; abstract S41.007.

37. Comi G, Kappos L, Palace J, et al. Cardiac safety of fingolimod 0.5 mg during the first dose observation in 4-month, open-label, multi-center FIRST study in patients with relapsing MS. Neurology 2012;78(suppl 1): S41.003.

38. Comi G, O'Connor P, Montalban X, et al. Phase II study of oral fingolimod (FTY720) in multiple sclerosis: 3-year results. Mult Scler 2010;16:197-207.

39. Food and Drug Administration. Gilenya (fingolimod): drug safety communication – safety review of a reported death after the first dose. December 12, 2011. Updated May 14, 2012. www.fda.gov/Safety/MedWatch/SafetyInformation/SafetyAlertsforHumanMedicalProducts/ucm284355.htm.

40. Novartis press release. Novartis statement on reported multiple sclerosis (MS) deaths of patients on Gilenya (fingolimod) from any cause through December 13, 2011. Updated March 13, 2012. www.novartis.com/downloads/newsroom/product-related-info-center/statement.pdf.

41. Food and Drug Administration. FDA Drug Safety Communication: Safety review of a reported death after the first dose of multiple sclerosis drug Gilenya (fingolimod). December 20, 2012. www.fda.gov/Drugs/DrugSafety/ucm284240.htm.

42. European Medicines Agency. European Medicines Agency gives new advice to better manage risk of adverse effects on the heart with Gilenya. www.ema.europa.eu/docs/en_GB/document_library/Press_release/2012/04/WC500125690.pdf.

43. Gilenya (fingolimod) Product Monograph. Revised April 2014. www.accessdata.fda.gov/drugsatfda_docs/label/2014/022527s009lbl.pdf

44. Gilenya (fingolimod) Product Monograph, February 12, 2014.

45. Novartis Pharmaceuticals Canada Inc. Health Canada endorsed important safety information on Gilenya (fingolimod). August 21, 2012. http://novartis.ca/products/en/pharmaceuticals-g.shtml.

46. Top 100 drugs for Q1 2013 by sales. www.drugs.com/stats/top100/sales.

47. Gilenya sales data. Updated May 2013. www.drugs.com/stats/gilenya.

48. Singer BA. Fingolimod for the treatment of relapsing multiple sclerosis. Expert Rev Neurother 2013;13:589-602.

49. Food and Drug Administration. Center for Drug Evaluation and Research. Medical review: Fingolimod. Application number: 22-527. August 26, 2010.

50. Miron VE, Schubart A, Antel JP. Central nervous system-directed effects of FTY720 (fingolimod). J Neurol Sci 2008;274:13-7.

51. Jung CG, Kim HJ, Miron VE, et al. Functional consequences of S1P receptor modulation in rat oligodendroglial lineage cells. Glia 2007;55:1656-67.

52. Miron VE, Jung CG, et al. FTY720 modulates human oligodendrocyte progenitor process extension and survival. Ann Neurol 2008;63:61-71.

53. Miron VE, Ludwin SK, Darlington PJ, et al. Fingolimod (FTY720) enhances remyelination following demyelination of organotypic cerebellar slices. Am J Pathol 2010;176:2682-94.

54. Jackson SJ, Giovannoni G, Baker D. Fingolimod modulates microglial activation to augment markers of remyelination. J Neuroinflammation 2011;8:76.

55. Zhang J, Zhang A, Sun Y, et al. Treatment with immunosuppressants FTY720 and tacrolimus promotes functional recovery after spinal cord injury in rats. Tohoku J Exp Med 2009;219:295-302.

56. Liu J, Zhang C, Tao W, Liu M. Systematic review and meta-analysis of the efficacy of sphingosine-1-phosphate (S1P) receptor agonist FTY720 (fingolimod) in animal models of stroke. Int J Neurosci 2013;123:163-9.

57. Novartis provides update on fingolimod Phase III trial in primary progressive MS (PPMS). Press release, December 1, 2014. www.novartis.com/newsroom/media-releases/en/2014/1875463.shtml.

58. Rinaldi F, Seppi D, Calabrese M, et al. Switching therapy from natalizumab to fingolimod in relapsing-remitting multiple sclerosis: clinical and magnetic resonance imaging findings. Mult Scler 2012;18:1640-3.

59. Sempere AP, Martín-Medina P, Berenguer-Ruiz L, et al. Switching from natalizumab to fingolimod: an observational study. Acta Neurol Scand 2013;128:e6-e10.

60. Depaz RR, Gueguen AA, Deschamps R, et al. Fingolimod initiation at the time of return of clinical activity following natalizumab cessation: short term outcome. Presented at the American Academy of Neurology annual meeting, San Diego CA, March 16- 23, 2013; abstract P01.208.

61. Havla J, Tackenberg B, Hellwig K, et al. Fingolimod reduces recurrence of disease activity after natalizumab withdrawal in multiple sclerosis. J Neurol 2013;260:1382-7.

62. Comi G, Gold R, Dahlke F, et al. Relapse outcomes in fingolimod-treated patients previously exposed to natalizumab: post-hoc analysis from the 4-month, open-label FIRST Study. Presented at the American Academy of Neurology annual meeting, San Diego CA, March 16- 23, 2013; abstract P07.103.

63. Putzki N, Clifford DB, Bischof D, et al. Characteristics of PML cases in multiple sclerosis patients switching to fingolimod from natalizumab. Presented at the joint

Americas and European Committee for Treatment and Research in Multiple Sclerosis (ACTRIMS-ECTRIMS) meeting, Boston, MA, September 10-13, 2014; abstract FC3.1.

64. Novartis. Gilenya safety update, February 16, 2015. www.novartis.com /newsroom/product-related-info-center/gilenya-safety-update.shtml.

CHAPTER 9. WHAT IS TECFIDERA?

1. Schweckendiek W. Treatment of psoriasis vulgaris. Med Monatsschr 1959;13:103-4.

2. Baati T, Horcajada P, Gref R, et al. Quantification of fumaric acid in liver, spleen and urine by high-performance liquid chromatography coupled to photodiode-array detection. J Pharm Biomed Anal 2011;56:758-62.

3. Nieboer C, de Hoop D, van Loenen AC, et al. Systemic therapy with fumaric acid derivates: new possibilities in the treatment of psoriasis. J Am Acad Dermatol 1989;20:601-8.

4. Raab W. Psoriasis therapy with fumaric acid and fumaric acid esters. Z Hautkr 1984;59:671-9.

5. de Haan P, von Blomberg-van der Flier BM, de Groot J, et al. The risk of sensibilization and contact urticaria upon topical application of fumaric acid derivatives. Dermatology 1994;188:126-30.

6. Bayard W, Hunziker T, Krebs A, et al. Peroral long-term treatment of psoriasis using fumaric acid derivatives. Hautarzt 1987;38:279-85.

7. Nieboer C, de Hoop D, Langendijk PN, et al. Fumaric acid therapy in psoriasis: a double-blind comparison between fumaric acid compound therapy and monotherapy with dimethylfumaric acid ester. Dermatologica 1990;181:33-7.

8. Nugteren-Huying WM, van der Schroeff JG, Hermans J, Suurmond D. Fumaric acid therapy in psoriasis; a double-blind, placebo-controlled study. Ned Tijdschr Geneeskd 1990;134:2387-91.

9. Altmeyer PJ, Matthes U, Pawlak F, et al. Antipsoriatic effect of fumaric acid derivatives. Results of a multicenter double-blind study in 100 patients. J Am Acad Dermatol 1994;30:977-81.

10. Mrowietz U, Christophers E, Altmeyer P. Treatment of psoriasis with fumaric acid esters: results of a prospective multicentre study. German Multicentre Study. Br J Dermatol 1998;138:456-60.

11. Moharregh-Khiabani D, Linker RA, Gold R, Stangel M. Fumaric acid and its esters: an emerging treatment for multiple sclerosis. Curr Neuropharmacol 2009;7:60-4.

12. Dethlefsen LA, Lehman CM, Biaglow JE, Peck VM. Toxic effects of acute glutathione depletion by buthionine sulfoximine and dimethylfumarate on murine mammary carcinoma cells. Radiat Res 1988;114:215-24.

13. Lehmann M, Risch K, Nizze H, et al. Fumaric acid esters are potent immunosuppressants: inhibition of acute and chronic rejection in rat kidney transplantation models by methyl hydrogen fumarate. Arch Dermatol Res 2002;294: 399-404.

14. Venten I, Hess N, Hirschmüller A, et al. Treatment of therapy-resistant alopecia areata with fumaric acid esters. Eur J Med Res 2006;11:300-5.

15. Treumer F, Zhu K, Gläser R, Mrowietz U. Dimethylfumarate is a potent inducer of apoptosis in human T cells. J Invest Dermatol 2003;121:1383-8.

16. Anon. BG 12: BG 00012, BG 12/Oral Fumarate, FAG-201, second-generation fumarate derivative--Fumapharm/Biogen Idec. Drugs R D 2005;6:229-30.

17. Biogen Idec press release. Biogen Idec to acquire Fumapharm AG; consolidates ownership of oral compound BG-12 being studied for multiple sclerosis. May 31, 2006. www.biogenidec.com/PRESS_RELEASE_DETAILS.aspx?ID= 5981&ReqId=862060.

18. Wakkee M, Thio HB. Drug evaluation: BG-12, an immunomodulatory dimethylfumarate. Curr Opin Investig Drugs 2007;8:955-62.

19. Tecfidera (dimethyl fumarate) Product Monograph. Revised March 2013.

20. Mrowietz U, Christophers E, Altmeyer P. Treatment of severe psoriasis with fumaric acid esters: scientific background and guidelines for therapeutic use. The German Fumaric Acid Ester Consensus Conference. Br J Dermatol 1999;141:424-9.

21. Litjens NHR, van Strijen E, van Gulpen C, et al. In vitro pharmacokinetics of anti-psoriatic fumaric acid esters. BMC Pharmacology 2004;4:22.

22. Litjens NH, Burggraaf J, van Strijen E, et al. Pharmacokinetics of oral fumarates in healthy subjects. Br J Clin Pharmacol 2004;58:429-32.

23. Vandermeeren M, Janssens S, Borgers M, Geysen J. Dimethylfumarate is an inhibitor of cytokine-induced E-selectin, VCAM-1, and ICAM-1 expression in human endothelial cells. Biochem Biophys Res Commun 1997;234:19-23.

24. Wallbrecht K, Drick N, Hund AC, Schön MP. Downregulation of endothelial adhesion molecules by dimethylfumarate, but not monomethylfumarate, and impairment of dynamic lymphocyte-endothelial cell interactions. Exp Dermatol 2011;20:980-5.

25. Litjens NH, Rademaker M, Ravensbergen B, et al. Effects of monomethylfumarate on dendritic cell differentiation. Br J Dermatol 2006;154:211-7.

26. de Jong R, Bezemer AC, Zomerdijk TP, et al. Selective stimulation of T helper 2 cytokine responses by the anti-psoriasis agent monomethylfumarate. Eur J Immunol 1996; 26:2067-74.

27. Lehmann JC, Listopad JJ, Rentzsch CU, et al. Dimethylfumarate induces immunosuppression via glutathione depletion and subsequent induction of heme oxygenase 1. J Invest Dermatol 2007;127:835-45.

28. Hoxtermann S, Nüchel C, Altmeyer P. Fumaric acid esters suppress peripheral CD4- and CD8-positive lymphocytes in psoriasis. Dermatology 1998;196:223-30.

29. Yan Z, Banerjee R. Redox remodeling as an immunoregulatory strategy. Biochemistry 2010; 49:1059.

30. Thoren FB, Betten A, Romero AI, Hellstrand K. Cutting edge: Antioxidative properties of myeloid dendritic cells: protection of T cells and NK cells from oxygen radical-induced inactivation and apoptosis. J Immunol 2007;179:21-5.

31. Gray E, Thomas TL, Betmouni S, et al. Elevated myeloperoxidase activity in white matter in multiple sclerosis. Neurosci Lett 2008;444:195-8.

32. Gray E, Thomas TL, Betmouni S, et al. Elevated activity and microglial expression of myeloperoxidase in demyelinated cerebral cortex in multiple sclerosis. Brain Pathol 2008;18:86-95.

33. Schmidt MM, Dringen R. Fumaric acid diesters deprive cultured primary astrocytes rapidly of glutathione. Neurochem Int 2010;57:460-7.

34. Thiessen A, Schmidt MM, Dringen R. Fumaric acid dialkyl esters deprive cultured rat oligodendroglial cells of glutathione and upregulate the expression of heme oxygenase 1. Neurosci Lett 2010;475:56-60.

35. Scannevin RH, Chollate S, Jung MY, et al. Fumarates promote cytoprotection of central nervous system cells against oxidative stress via the nuclear factor (erythroid-derived 2)-like 2 pathway. J Pharmacol Exp Ther 2012;341:274-84.

36. Lin SX, Lisi L, Dello Russo C, et al The anti-inflammatory effects of dimethyl fumarate in astrocytes involve glutathione and haem oxygenase-1. ASN Neuro 2011;3.

37. Jiang J, Mo ZC, Yin K, et al. Epigallocatechin-3-gallate prevents TNF-α-induced NF-κB activation thereby upregulating ABCA1 via the Nrf2/Keap1 pathway in macrophage foam cells. Int J Mol Med 2012;29:946-56.

38. Gerdes S, Shakery K, Mrowietz U. Dimethylfumarate inhibits nuclear binding of nuclear factor kappaB but not of nuclear factor of activated T cells and CCAAT/enhancer binding protein beta in activated human T cells. Br J Dermatol 2007;156:838-42.

39. Loewe R, Holnthoner W, Gröger M, et al. Dimethylfumarate inhibits TNF-induced nuclear entry of NF-kappa B/p65 in human endothelial cells.J Immunol 2002;168:4781-7.

40. Liu GH, Qu J, Shen X. NF-kappaB/p65 antagonizes Nrf2-ARE pathway by depriving CBP from Nrf2 and facilitating recruitment of HDAC3 to MafK. Biochim Biophys Acta 2008;1783:713-27.

41. Schimrigk S, Brune N, Hellwig K, et al. Oral fumaric acid esters for the treatment of active multiple sclerosis: an open-label, baseline-controlled pilot study. Eur J Neurol 2006;13:604-10.

42. Kappos L, Gold R, Miller DH, et al. Efficacy and safety of oral fumarate in patients with relapsing-remitting multiple sclerosis: a multicentre, randomised, double-blind, placebo-controlled phase IIb study. Lancet 2008;372:1463-72.

43. Rantanen T. The cause of the Chinese sofa/chair dermatitis epidemic is likely to be contact allergy to dimethylfumarate, a novel potent contact sensitizer. Br J Dermatol 2008;159:218-21.

44. Susitaival P, Winhoven SM, Williams J, et al. An outbreak of furniture related dermatitis ('sofa dermatitis') in Finland and the UK: history and clinical cases. J Eur Acad Dermatol Venereol 2010;24:486-9.

45. Lefranc A, Flesch F, Cochet A, et al. Epidemiological description of an outbreak of dermatitis related to dimethylfumarate, France, 2008. Arch Environ Occup Health 2011;66:217-22.

46. Foti C, Zambonin CG, Cassano N, et al. Occupational allergic contact dermatitis associated with dimethyl fumarate in clothing. Contact Dermatitis 2009;61:122-4.

47. Giménez-Arnau A, Silvestre JF, Mercader P, et al. Shoe contact dermatitis from dimethyl fumarate: clinical manifestations, patch test results, chemical analysis, and source of exposure. Contact Dermatitis 2009;61:249-60.

48. Pastor-Nieto MA, Quintanilla-López JE, Gómara B, et al. Contact dermatitis caused by dimethyl fumarate in wallets. Contact Dermatitis 2013;68:118-20.

49. Stefanelli P, Girolimetti S, Santilio A, Dommarco R. Survey of dimethyl fumarate in desiccant products during 2009 in Italy. Bull Environ Contam Toxicol 2011;86:428-32.

50. Ropper AH. The "poison chair" treatment for multiple sclerosis. N Engl J Med 2012;367:1149-50.

51. Gold R, Kappos L, Arnold DL, et al. Placebo-controlled phase 3 study of oral BG-12 for relapsing multiple sclerosis. N Engl J Med 2012;367:1098-107.

52. Kita M, Fox R, Phillips T, et al. Clinical and neuroradiologic efficacy of BG-12 (dimethyl fumarate) in US patients with relapsing-remitting multiple sclerosis (RRMS): An integrated analysis of the phase 3 DEFINE and CONFIRM studies. Presented at the American Academy of Neurology annual meeting, San Diego CA, March 16-23, 2013; abstract P07.091.

53. Food and Drug Administration. Center for Drug Evaluation and Research. Tecfidera Summary Review, February 11, 2013.

54. Hoefnagel JJ, Thio HB, Willemze R, et al. Long-term safety aspects of systemic therapy with fumaric acid esters in severe psoriasis. Br J Dermatol 2003;149:363-9.

55. Jennings L, Murphy G. Squamous cell carcinoma as a complication of fumaric acid ester immunosuppression. J Eur Acad Dermatol Venereol 2009;23:1451.

56. Barth D, Simon JC, Wetzig T. Malignant melanoma during treatment with fumaric acid esters - coincidence or treatment-related? J Dtsch Dermatol Ges 2011;9:223-5.

57. Roodnat JI, Christiaans MH, Nugteren-Huying WM, et al. Acute kidney insufficiency in the treatment of psoriasis using fumaric esters. Schweiz Med Wochenschr 1989;119:826-30.

58. Raschka C, Koch HJ. Longterm treatment of psoriasis using fumaric acid preparations can be associated with severe proximal tubular damage. Hum Exp Toxicol 1999;18:738-39.

59. Fox RJ, Miller DH, Phillips JT, et al. Placebo-controlled phase 3 study of oral BG-12 or glatiramer in multiple sclerosis.N Engl J Med 2012;367:1087-97.

60. Fox RJ, Havrdova E. Oral BG-12 in multiple sclerosis. N Engl J Med 2013;17:1652-1653.

61. Tecfidera (dimethyl fumarate) Product Monograph, March 2013.

62. Tecfidera (dimethyl fumarate) Canadian Product Monograph, March 28, 2013.

63. Health Canada. Tecfidera: Summary Basic of Decision, May 27, 2013. www.hc-sc.gc.ca/dhp-mps/prodpharma/sbd-smd/drug-med/sbd_smd_2013_tecfidera_154776-eng.php.

64. Sweetser MT, Dawson KT, Bozic C. Manufacturer's response to case reports of PML. N Engl J Med 2013;368:1659-61.

65. Food and Drug Administration. FDA Drug Safety Communication: FDA warns about case of rare brain infection PML with MS drug Tecfidera (dimethyl fumarate). November 25, 2014. www.fda.gov/Drugs/DrugSafety/ucm424625.htm. Accessed February 8, 2015.

66. Pozzilli C, Phillips JT, Fox RJ, et al. Long-term follow-up of the safety of delayed-release dimethyl fumarate in RRMS: interim results from the ENDORSE extension study. Presented at the joint Americas and European Committee for Treatment and Research in Multiple Sclerosis (ACTRIMS-ECTRIMS) meeting, Boston, MA, September 10-13, 2014; abstract P066.

67. Molloy ES1, Calabrese LH. Progressive multifocal leukoencephalopathy associated with immunosuppressive therapy in rheumatic diseases: evolving role of biologic therapies. Arthritis Rheum 2012;64:3043-3051.

68. Tecfidera (dimethyl fumarate) Product Monograph. Revised December 3, 2014.

69. Phillips JT, Hutchinson M, Fox R, et al. Management strategies for flushing and gastrointestinal events associated with BG-12 (dimethyl fumarate): expert panel recommendations. Presented at the 29th Congress of the European Committee for Treatment and Research in Multiple Sclerosis, Copenhagen, Denmark, October 2-5, 2013; abstract P549.

70. Tornatore C, Li J, Ma T, et al. Effect of bismuth subsalicylate on gastrointestinal events associated with delayed-release dimethyl fumarate: a double-blind, placebo-controlled study. Presented at the joint Americas and European Committee for Treatment and Research in Multiple Sclerosis (ACTRIMS-ECTRIMS) meeting, Boston, MA, September 10-13, 2014; abstract P052.

71. Fox EJ, Vasquez A, Grainger W, et al. Gastrointestinal tolerability of delayed-release dimethyl fumarate in a multicenter, open-label study of patients with relapsing multiple sclerosis. Presented at the joint Americas and European Committee for Treatment and Research in Multiple Sclerosis (ACTRIMS-ECTRIMS) meeting, Boston, MA, September 10-13, 2014; abstract P309.

72. Gold R, Giovannoni G, Phillips JT, et al. Long-term efficacy of delayed-release dimethyl fumarate in newly diagnosed patients with RRMS: an integrated analysis of DEFINE, CONFIRM, and ENDORSE. Presented at the joint Americas and European Committee for Treatment and Research in Multiple Sclerosis (ACTRIMS-ECTRIMS) meeting, Boston, MA, September 10-13, 2014; abstract P064.

73. Selmaj K, Gold R, Fox RJ, et al. Flushing and gastrointestinal tolerability events in relapsing remitting multiple sclerosis (RRMS) patients treated with oral BG-12 dimethyl fumarate) in the phase 3 DEFINE and CONFIRM trials. Presented at the 29th Congress of the European Committee for Treatment and Research in Multiple Sclerosis, Copenhagen, Denmark, October 2-5, 2013; abstract P537.

CHAPTER 10. WHAT IS AUBAGIO?

1. Bartlett RR, Schleyerbach R. Immunopharmacological profile of a novel isoxazol derivative, HWA 486, with potential antirheumatic activity--I. Disease modifying action on adjuvant arthritis of the rat. Int J Immunopharmacol 1985;7:7-18.

2. Bartlett RR, Dimitrijevic M, Mattar T, et al. Leflunomide (HWA 486), a novel immunomodulating compound for the treatment of autoimmune disorders and reactions leading to transplantation rejection. Agents Actions 1991;32:10-21.

3. Vidic-Dankovic B, Kosec D, Damjanovic M, et al. Leflunomide prevents the development of experimentally induced myasthenia gravis. Int J Immunopharmacol 1995;17:273-81.

4. van Woerkom JM, Kruize AA, Geenen R, et al. Safety and efficacy of leflunomide in primary Sjögren's syndrome: a phase II pilot study. Ann Rheum Dis 2007;66:1026-32.

5. Chong AS, Finnegan A, Jiang X, et al. Leflunomide, a novel immunosuppressive agent. The mechanism of inhibition of T cell proliferation. Transplantation 1993;55:1361-6.

6. Zielinski T, Müller HJ, Bartlett RR. Effects of leflunomide (HWA 486) on expression of lymphocyte activation markers. Agents Actions 1993;38 Spec No:C80-2.

7. Cao WW, Kao PN, Chao AC, et al. Mechanism of the antiproliferative action of leflunomide. A77 1726, the active metabolite of leflunomide, does not block T-cell

receptor-mediated signal transduction but its antiproliferative effects are antagonized by pyrimidine nucleosides. J Heart Lung Transplant 1995;14(6 Pt 1):1016-30.

8. Xu X, Williams JW, Gong H, et al. Two activities of the immunosuppressive metabolite of leflunomide, A77 1726. Inhibition of pyrimidine nucleotide synthesis and protein tyrosine phosphorylation. Biochem Pharmacol 1996;52:527-34.

9. Baldwin J, Farajallah AM, Malmquist NA, et al. Malarial dihydroorotate dehydrogenase. Substrate and inhibitor specificity. J Biol Chem 2002;277:41827-34.

10. Manna SK, Aggarwal BB. Immunosuppressive leflunomide metabolite (A77 1726) blocks TNF-dependent nuclear factor-kappa B activation and gene expression. J Immunol 1999;162:2095-102.

11. Kobayashi Y, Ueyama S, Arai Y, et al. The active metabolite of leflunomide, A771726, inhibits both the generation of and the bone-resorbing activity of osteoclasts by acting directly on cells of the osteoclast lineage. J Bone Miner Metab 2004;22:318-28.

12. Miljkovic D, Samardzic T, Mostarica Stojkovic M, et al. Leflunomide inhibits activation of inducible nitric oxide synthase in rat astrocytes. Brain Res 2001;889:331-8.

13. Reuters. UPDATE-1 – Sanofi's MS drugs get double boost in Europe. June 28, 2013.

14. O'Connor PW, Li D, Freedman MS, et al. A phase II study of the safety and efficacy of teriflunomide in multiple sclerosis with relapses. Neurology 2006;66:894-900.

15. Food and Drug Administration. Center for Drug Evaluation and Research. Teriflunomide: Clinical pharmacology and biopharmaceutics review(s). September 28, 2011.

16. Confavreux C, Li D, Freedman M, et al. Long-term follow-up of a phase 2 study of oral teriflunomide in relapse multiple sclerosis: safety and efficacy results up to 8.5 years. Mult Scler 2012;18:1278-89.

17. O'Connor P, Wolinsky JS, Confavreux C, et al. Randomized trial of oral teriflunomide for relapsing multiple sclerosis. N Engl J Med 2011;365:1293-303.

18. Food and Drug Administration. Center for Drug Evaluation and Research. Teriflunomide: Summary review. July 27, 2012.

19. Freedman M, Wolinsky J, Comi G, et al. Long-term safety and efficacy of teriflunomide in patients with relapsing forms of multiple sclerosis in the TEMSO extension trial. Presented at the 29th Congress of the European Committee for Treatment and Research in Multiple Sclerosis, Copenhagen, Denmark, October 2-5, 2013; abstract P544.

20. Confavreux C, O'Connor P, Comi G, et al. Oral teriflunomide for patients with relapsing multiple sclerosis (TOWER): a randomised, double-blind, placebo-controlled, phase 3 trial. Lancet Neurol 2014;13:247-256.

21. Miller A, Wolinsky J, Kappos L, et al. TOPIC main outcomes: efficacy and safety of once-daily oral teriflunomide in patients with clinically isolated syndrome. Presented at the 29th Congress of the European Committee for Treatment and Research in Multiple Sclerosis, Copenhagen, Denmark, October 2-5, 2013; abstract 99.

22. Vermersch P, Czlonkowska A, Grimaldi LM, et al. Teriflunomide versus subcutaneous interferon beta-1a in patients with relapsing multiple sclerosis: a

randomised, controlled phase 3 trial. Mult Scler 2013; epublished November 21, 2013.

23. Kappos L, Comi G, Freedman MS, et al. Pooled safety data from three placebo-controlled teriflunomide studies. Presented at the 29th Congress of the European Committee for Treatment and Research in Multiple Sclerosis, Copenhagen, Denmark, October 2-5, 2013; abstract P618.

24. Kieseier B, Benamor M, Truffinet P, Henson LJ. Pregnancy outcomes for female patients and partners of male patients in the teriflunomide clinical development program. Presented at the joint Americas and European Committee for Treatment and Research in Multiple Sclerosis (ACTRIMS-ECTRIMS) meeting, Boston, MA, September 10-13, 2014; abstract P846.

25. Anonymous . Phase II study of teriflunomide as adjunctive therapy to glatiramer acetate in subjects with multiple sclerosis. NCT00475865. Clinicaltrials.gov. Accessed June 2, 2013.

26. Freedman MS, Wolinsky JS, Wamil B, et al. Teriflunomide added to interferon-β in relapsing multiple sclerosis: a randomized phase II trial. Neurology 2012;78:1877-85.

27. Freedman MS, Wamil BD, Cheng S, et al. TERACLES study design: teriflunomide as adjunctive therapy in patients with relapsing multiple sclerosis receiving interferon beta. Presented at the Fifth Cooperative meeting of the Consortium of Multiple Sclerosis Centers (CMSC) and Americas Committee for Treatment and Research in Multiple Sclerosis (ACTRIMS) meeting. Orlando FL, May 29-June 1, 2013.

CHAPTER 11. WHAT IS LEMTRADA?

1. Schwaber J, Cohen EP. Human x mouse somatic cell hybrid clone secreting immunoglobulins of both parental types. Nature 1973;244:444-7.

2. Köhler G, Milstein C. Continuous cultures of fused cells secreting antibody of predefined specificity. Nature 1975;256:495-7.

3. Waldmann H, Hale G. CAMPATH: from concept to clinic. Phil Trans R Soc B 2005;360:1707-11.

4. Xia MQ, Tone M, Packman L, et al. Characterization of the CAMPATH-1 (CDw52) antigen: biochemical analysis and cDNA cloning reveal an unusually small peptide backbone. Eur J Immunol 1991;21:1677-84.

5. Hale G, Waldmann H. From laboratory to clinic: the story of CAMPATH-1. In George AJT, Urch CE, eds. Diagnostic and Therapeutic Antibodies. Totowa NJ: Humana Press, 2000. http://users.path.ox.ac.uk/~scobbold/tig/campath/camphist.htm. Accessed June 21, 2013.

6. Moreau T, Coles A, Wing M, et al. CAMPATH-IH in multiple sclerosis. Mult Scler 1996;1:357-65.

7. Moreau T, Coles A, Wing MG, et al. Transient increase in symptoms associated with cytokine release in patients with multiple sclerosis Brain 1996;119:225-37.

8. Coles AJ, Wing M, Smith S, et al. Pulsed monoclonal antibody treatment and autoimmune thyroid disease in multiple sclerosis. Lancet 1999;354:1691-5.

9. Coles AJ, Wing MG, Molyneux P, et al. Monoclonal antibody treatment exposes three mechanisms underlying the clinical course of multiple sclerosis. Ann Neurol 1999;46:296-304.

10. Coles AJ, Wing M, Smith S, et al. Pulsed monoclonal antibody treatment and autoimmune thyroid disease in multiple sclerosis. Lancet 1999;354:1691-5.

11. Hill-Cawthorne GA, Button T, Tuohy O, et al. Long term lymphocyte reconstitution after alemtuzumab treatment of multiple sclerosis. J Neurol Neurosurg Psychiatry 2012;83:298-304.

12. Paolillo A, Coles AJ, Molyneux PD, et al. Quantitative MRI in patients with secondary progressive MS treated with monoclonal antibody Campath 1H. Neurology 1999;53:751-7.

13. Hirst CL, Pace A, Pickersgill TP, et al. Campath 1-H treatment in patients with aggressive relapsing remitting multiple sclerosis. J Neurol 2008;255:231-8.

14. CAMMS223 Trial Investigators, Coles AJ, Compston DA, et al. Alemtuzumab vs. interferon beta-1a in early multiple sclerosis. N Engl J Med 2008;359:1786-801.

15. Jones JL, Anderson JM, Phuah CL, et al. Improvement in disability after alemtuzumab treatment of multiple sclerosis is associated with neuroprotective autoimmunity. Brain 2010;133(Pt 8):2232-47.

16. Coles AJ, Fox E, Vladic A, et al. Alemtuzumab more effective than interferon β-1a at 5-year follow-up of CAMMS223 clinical trial. Neurology 2012;78:1069-78.

17. Martin SI, Marty FM, Fiumara K, et al. Infectious complications associated with alemtuzumab use for lymphoproliferative disorders. Clin Infect Dis 2006;43:16-24.

18. Waggoner J, Martinu T, Palmer SM. Progressive multifocal leukoencephalopathy following heightened immunosuppression after lung transplant. J Heart Lung Transplant 2009;28:395-8.

19. Keene DL, Legare C, Taylor E, et al. Monoclonal antibodies and progressive multifocal leukoencephalopathy. Can J Neurol Sci 2011;38:565-71.

20. Anon. Alemtuzumab for multiple sclerosis. Lancet 2012;380:1792.

21. Cohen JA, Coles AJ, Arnold DL, et al. Alemtuzumab versus interferon beta 1a as first-line treatment for patients with relapsing-remitting multiple sclerosis: a randomised controlled phase 3 trial. Lancet 2012;380:1819-28.

22. Coles AJ, Twyman CL, Arnold DL, et al. Alemtuzumab for patients with relapsing multiple sclerosis after disease-modifying therapy: a randomised controlled phase 3 trial. Lancet 2012;380:1829-39.

23. Hartung H-P, Arnold DL, Cohen JA, et al. Efficacy and safety of alemtuzumab in patients with relapsing-remitting MS who relapsed on prior therapy: four-year follow-up of the CARE-MS II study. Presented at the joint Americas and European Committee for Treatment and Research in Multiple Sclerosis (ACTRIMS-ECTRIMS) meeting, Boston, MA, September 10-13, 2014; abstract P043.

24. Food and Drug Administration (FDA). Center for Drug Evaluation and Research (CDER) Peripheral and Central Nervous System Drugs Advisory Committee Meeting. Alemtuzumab (BLA 103948\5139): Background Package. November 13, 2013. www.fda.gov/downloads/AdvisoryCommittees/ CommitteesMeeting Materials/Drugs/PeripheralandCentralNervousSystemDrugsAdvisoryCommittee/ UCM374186.pdf. Accessed November 14, 2013.

25. European Medicines Agency. European Public Assessment Report, September 25, 2013. www.ema.europa.eu/ema/index.jsp?curl=/pages/medicines/human/ medicines/ 003718/human_med_001678.jsp. Accessed November 14, 2013.

26. Bennett S, Tirrell M. Sanofi MS Drug's Mixed Verdict From FDA Panel Puzzles Analysts. Bloomberg, November 14, 2013. www.bloomberg.com/news/2013-11-

14/sanofi-ms-drug-s-mixed-verdict-from-fda-panel-puzzles-analysts.html. Accessed November 14, 2013.

CHAPTER 12. HOW DO I CHOOSE A THERAPY?

1. Scalfari A, Neuhaus A, Degenhardt A, et al. The natural history of multiple sclerosis, a geographically based study 10: relapses and long-term disability. Brain 2010;133:1914-29.

2. Tremlett H, Zhao Y, Joseph J, et al. Relapses in multiple sclerosis are age and time dependent. J Neurol Neurosurg Psychiatry 2008;79:1368-74.

3. Mowry EM, Pesic M, Grimes B, et al. Demyelinating events in early multiple sclerosis have inherent severity and recovery. Neurology 2009;72:602-8.

4. Langer-Gould A, Popat RA, Huang SM, et al. Clinical and demographic predictors of long-term disability in patients with relapsing-remitting multiple sclerosis: a systematic review. Arch Neurol 2006;63:1686-91.

5. Rudick RA, Lee JC, Simon J, et al. Defining interferon beta response status in multiple sclerosis patients. Ann Neurol 2004;56:548-55.

6. Tremlett H, Yousefi M, Devonshire V, et al. Impact of multiple sclerosis relapses on progression diminishes with time. Neurology 2009;73:1616-23.

7. Lugaresi A, di Ioia M, Travaglini D, Pietrolongo E, Pucci E, Onofrj M. Risk-benefit considerations in the treatment of relapsing-remitting multiple sclerosis. Neuropsychiatr Dis Treat 2013;9:893-914.

8. Mikol DD, Barkhof F, Chang P, et al. Comparison of subcutaneous interferon beta-1a with glatiramer acetate in patients with relapsing multiple sclerosis (the REbif vs Glatiramer Acetate in Relapsing MS Disease [REGARD] study): a multicentre, randomised, parallel, open-label trial. Lancet Neurol 2008;7:903-14.

9. Cadavid D, Wolansky LJ, Skurnick J, et al. Efficacy of treatment of MS with IFNbeta-1b or glatiramer acetate by monthly brain MRI in the BECOME study. Neurology 2009;72:1976-83.

10. O'Connor P, Filippi M, Arnason B, et al. 250 microg or 500 microg interferon beta-1b versus 20 mg glatiramer acetate in relapsing-remitting multiple sclerosis: a prospective, randomised, multicentre study. Lancet Neurol 2009;8:889-97.

11. Beer K, Muller M, Hew-Winzeler AM, et al. The prevalence of injection-site reactions with disease-modifying therapies and their effect on adherence in patients with multiple sclerosis: an observational study. BMC Neurol 2011;11:144.

12. IFNB Multiple Sclerosis Study Group. Interferon beta-1b in the treatment of multiple sclerosis: final outcome of the randomized controlled trial. Neurology 1995;45:1277-85.

13. Evans C, Tam J, Kingwell E, et al. Long-term persistence with the immunomodulatory drugs for multiple sclerosis: a retrospective database study. Clin Ther 2012;34:341-50.

14. Wong J, Gomes T, Mamdani M, et al. Adherence to multiple sclerosis disease-modifying therapies in Ontario is low. Can J Neurol Sci 2011;38:429-33.

15. Portaccio E, Zipoli V, Siracusa G, et al. Long-term adherence to interferon beta therapy in relapsing-remitting multiple sclerosis. Eur Neurol 2008;59:131-5.

16. Steinberg SC, Faris RJ, Chang CF, et al. Impact of adherence to interferons in the treatment of multiple sclerosis: a non-experimental, retrospective, cohort study. Clin Drug Investig 2010;30:89-100.

17. Patti F. Optimizing the benefit of multiple sclerosis therapy: the importance of treatment adherence. Patient Prefer Adherence 2010;4:1-9.

18. Meyniel C, Spelman T, Jokubaitis VG, et al. Country, sex, EDSS change and therapy choice independently predict treatment discontinuation in multiple sclerosis and clinically isolated syndrome. PLoS One 2012;7:e38661.

19. Fox RJ. In the coming year we should abandon interferons and glatiramer acetate as first-line therapy for MS: Yes. Mult Scler 2013;19: 24-5.

20. Manners S. The Year in (P)review - MS 2013 – Is the Injectable Era (almost) Over? NeuroSens, January 31, 2013.

21. Vermersch P, Czlonkowska A, Grimaldi L, et al. Evaluation of patient satisfaction from the TENERE study: a comparison of teriflunomide and subcutaneous interferon beta-1a in patients with relapsing multiple sclerosis. Presented at the 23rd meeting of the European Neurological Society, Barcelona, Spain, June 8-11, 2013.

22. Fox RJ, Miller DH, Phillips JT, et al. Placebo-controlled phase 3 study of oral BG-12 or glatiramer in multiple sclerosis. N Engl J Med 2012;367:1087-97.

23. Healy BC, Glanz BI, Stankiewicz J, et al. A method for evaluating treatment switching criteria in multiple sclerosis. Mult Scler 2010;16:1483-9.

24. Freedman MS, Selchen D, Arnold DL, et al. Treatment optimization in MS: Canadian MS Working Group updated recommendations. Can J Neurol Sci 2013;40:307-23.

25. Pozzilli C, Prosperini L, Sbardella E, et al. Post-marketing survey on clinical response to interferon beta in relapsing multiple sclerosis: the Roman experience. Neurol Sci 2005;26 Suppl 4:S174-8.

26. Tomassini V, Paolillo A, Russo P, et al. Predictors of long-term clinical response to interferon beta therapy in relapsing multiple sclerosis. J Neurol 2006;253:287-93.

27. Prosperini L, Gallo V, Petsas N, et al. One-year MRI scan predicts clinical response to interferon beta in multiple sclerosis. Eur J Neurol 2009;16:1202-9.

28. Rio J, Rovira A, Tintore M, et al. Relationship between MRI lesion activity and response to IFN-beta in relapsing-remitting multiple sclerosis patients. Mult Scler 2008;14:479-84.

29. Cohen JA, Barkhof F, Comi G, et al. Oral fingolimod or intramuscular interferon for relapsing multiple sclerosis. N Engl J Med 2010;362:402-15.

30. Polman CH, O'Connor PW, Havrdova E, et al. Randomized, placebo-controlled trial of natalizumab for relapsing multiple sclerosis. N Engl J Med 2006;354:899-910.

31. Cohen JA, Coles AJ, Arnold DL, et al. Alemtuzumab versus interferon beta 1a as first-line treatment for patients with relapsing-remitting multiple sclerosis: a randomised controlled phase 3 trial. Lancet 2012;380:1819-28.

32. Coles AJ, Twyman CL, Arnold DL, et al. Alemtuzumab for patients with relapsing multiple sclerosis after disease-modifying therapy: a randomised controlled phase 3 trial. Lancet 2012;380:1829-39.

33. Prosperini L, Mancinelli CR, De Giglio L, et al. Interferon beta failure predicted by EMA criteria or isolated MRI activity in multiple sclerosis. Mult Scler 2013; epublished September 3, 2013.

34. Hohol MJ, Orav EJ, Weiner HL. Disease Steps in multiple sclerosis: A simple approach to evaluate disease progression. Neurology 1995;45:251-255. Available at www.narcoms.org/files/PDDS_Letter_111512_Final.pdf.

35. Hohol MJ, Orav EJ, Weiner HL. Disease Steps in multiple sclerosis: a longitudinal study comparing disease steps and EDSS to evaluate disease progression. Multiple Sclerosis 1999;5:349-54.

36. Miller AE, O'Connor P, Wolinsky JS, et al. Pre-specified subgroup analyses of a placebo-controlled phase III trial (TEMSO) of oral teriflunomide in relapsing multiple sclerosis. Mult Scler 2012;18:1625-32.

37. Kita M, Fox R, Phillips T, et al. Clinical and neuroradiologic efficacy of BG-12 (dimethyl fumarate) in US patients with relapsing-remitting multiple sclerosis (RRMS): An integrated analysis of the phase 3 DEFINE and CONFIRM studies. Presented at the American Academy of Neurology annual meeting, San Diego CA, March 16-23, 2013; abstract P07.091.

38. Castillo-Trivino T, Mowry EM, Gajofatto A, et al. Switching multiple sclerosis patients with breakthrough disease to second-line therapy. PLoS One 2011;6:e16664a

39. Putzki N, Yaldizli O, Maurer M, et al. Efficacy of natalizumab in second line therapy of relapsing-remitting multiple sclerosis: results from a multi-center study in German speaking countries. Eur J Neurol 2010;17:31-7.

40. Jokubaitis VG, Spelman T, Lechner-Scott J, et al. The Australian Multiple Sclerosis (MS) immunotherapy study: a prospective, multicentre study of drug utilisation using the MSBase platform. PLoS One 2013;8:e59694.

41. Cohen JA, Barkhof F, Comi G, et al. Oral fingolimod or intramuscular interferon for relapsing multiple sclerosis. N Engl J Med 2010;362:402-15.

42. Khatri B, Barkhof F, Comi G, et al. Comparison of fingolimod with interferon beta-1a in relapsing-remitting multiple sclerosis: a randomised extension of the TRANSFORMS study. Lancet Neurol 2011;10:520-9.

43. Comi G, Gold R, Kappos L, et al. Relapse and safety outcomes in patients who transitioned from glatiramer acetate or interferon beta to fingolimod in the open-label FIRST study. Presented at the 29th Congress of the European Committee for Treatment and Research in Multiple Sclerosis, Copenhagen, Denmark, October 2-5, 2013; abstract P513.

44. Spelman T, Bergvall N, Tomic D, et al. Real-world comparative effectiveness of fingolimod and interferon/glatiramer therapies in a switch population using propensity-matched data from MSBase. Presented at the 29th Congress of the European Committee for Treatment and Research in Multiple Sclerosis, Copenhagen, Denmark, October 2-5, 2013; abstract P1096.

45. Cree BAC, Kanton D, Steingo BM, et al. Patient- and physician-reported outcomes after therapy switch from glatiramer acetate to fingolimod versus staying on glatiramer acetate. Presented at the 29th Congress of the European Committee for Treatment and Research in Multiple Sclerosis, Copenhagen, Denmark, October 2-5, 2013; abstract P1010.

46. Bergvall N, Lahoz R, Agashivala N, et al. et al. Relapse rates among patients with a history of relapses treated with fingolimod compared with interferons or glatiramer acetate for the treatment of multiple sclerosis: a retrospective US claims database analysis. Presented at the 29th Congress of the European Committee for Treatment and Research in Multiple Sclerosis, Copenhagen, Denmark, October 2-5, 2013; abstract P637.

47. Edwards KR, Crayton H, Calkwood J, et al. Patient- and physician-reported outcomes after therapy switch from interferon beta to fingolimod versus staying on

interferon beta therapy. Presented at the 29th Congress of the European Committee for Treatment and Research in Multiple Sclerosis, Copenhagen, Denmark, October 2-5, 2013; abstract P555.

48. Braune S, Lang M, Bergmann A, et al. Second line use of fingolimod is as effective as natalizumab in a German out-patient RRMS cohort. J Neurol 2013;260:2981-2985.

49. Havrdova E, Galetta S, Hutchinson M, et al. Effect of natalizumab on clinical and radiological disease activity in multiple sclerosis: a retrospective analysis of the Natalizumab Safety and Efficacy in Relapsing-Remitting Multiple Sclerosis (AFFIRM) study. Lancet Neurol 2009;8:254-60.

50. Khatri B, Barkhof F, Comi G, et al. Fingolimod treatment increases the proportion of patients who are free from disease activity in multiple sclerosis compared to IFN-B1a: results from a phase 3, active-controlled study (TRANSFORMS). Neurology 2012;78(suppl 1): PD5.

51. Hartung H, Vollmer T, Arnold D, et al. Alemtuzumab reduces MS disease activity in active relapsing-remitting multiple sclerosis patients who had disease activity on prior therapy. Presented at the American Academy of Neurology annual meeting, San Diego CA, March 16- 23, 2013; abstract P07.093.

52. Kappos L, Radue E-W, O'Connor P, et al. Fingolimod treatment increases the proportion of patients who are free from disease activity in multiple sclerosis: results from a phase 3, placebo-controlled study (FREEDOMS). Presented at the 63rd annual meeting of the American Academy of Neurology, Honolulu HI, April 9-16, 2011; abstract PD6.002.

53. Perumal J, Khan O. Emerging disease-modifying therapies in multiple sclerosis. Curr Treat Options Neurol 2012;14:256-63.

54. Fazekas F, Bajenaru O, Berger T, et al. How does fingolimod (Gilenya(®)) fit in the treatment algorithm for highly active relapsing-remitting multiple sclerosis? Front Neurol 2013;4:10.

55. Ontaneda D, Hara-Cleaver C, Rudick RA, et al. Early tolerability and safety of fingolimod in clinical practice. J Neurol Sci 2012;323:167-72.

56. Maciejek Z, Wójcik-Drączkowska H, Wawrzyniak S, et al. Evaluation of efficacy, safety and tolerability of fingolimod in patients with the relapsing form of multiple sclerosis - 12-month observation. A preliminary report. Neurol Neurochir Pol 2013;47:145-51.

57. Piehl F, Holmen C, Hillert J, Olsson T. Swedish natalizumab (Tysabri) multiple sclerosis surveillance study. Neurol Sci 2011;31 Suppl 3:289-93.

58. Bloomgren G, Richman S, Hotermans C, et al. Risk of natalizumab-associated progressive multifocal leukoencephalopathy. N Engl J Med 2012;366:1870-80.

59. Biogen Idec, data on file, September 2013.

60. Frisullo et al. CD4+T-bet+, CD4+pSTAT3+ and CD8+T-bet+ T cells accumulate in peripheral blood during NZB treatment. Mult Scler 2011;17:556-66.

61. Kivisakk et al. Natalizumab treatment is associated with peripheral sequestration of proinflammatory T cells Neurology 2009;72:1922-30.

62. O'Connor PW, Goodman A, Kappos L, et al. Disease activity return during natalizumab treatment interruption in patients with multiple sclerosis. Neurology 2011;76:1858-65.

63. Clerico et al. Natalizumab discontinuation after the 24th course: Which is way? The TY-STOP study. Presented at the American Academy of Neurology annual meeting, San Diego CA, March 16- 23, 2013; abstract P01.197.

64. Borriello G, Prosperini L, Mancinelli C, et al. Pulse monthly steroids during an elective interruption of natalizumab: a post-marketing study. Eur J Neurol 2012;19:783-7.

65. Magraner MJ, Coret F, Navarré A, et al. Pulsed steroids followed by glatiramer acetate to prevent inflammatory activity after cessation of natalizumab therapy: a prospective, 6-month observational study. J Neurol 2011;258:1805-11.

66. Havla J, Tackenberg B, Hellwig K, et al. Fingolimod reduces recurrence of disease activity after natalizumab withdrawal in multiple sclerosis. J Neurol 2013;260:1382-7.

67. Kappos L, Radue EW, Comi G, et al. Disease control and safety in relapsing-remitting multiple sclerosis (RRMS) patients switching from natalizumab to fingolimod: a 32-week, rater- and patient-blind, randomized, parallel-group study (TOFINGO). Presented at the 29th Congress of the European Committee for Treatment and Research in Multiple Sclerosis, Copenhagen, Denmark, October 2-5, 2013; abstract 167.

68. Comi G. Algorithms. Presented at the 21st annual meeting of the European Charcot Foundation, Baveno, Italy, November 28-30, 2013.

69. Zarbin MA, Jampol LM, Jager RD, et al. Ophthalmic evaluations in clinical studies of fingolimod (FTY720) in multiple sclerosis. Ophthalmology 2013;120:1432-1439.

ACKNOWLEDGEMENTS

I would like to thank Anne St-Michel, publisher of *MSology* and *NeuroSens*, for her unfailing encouragement and support. Thanks also to Kate Stella for keeping the news services running as they should, and to INM for their excellent website design and technical support. I would also like to acknowledge and thank the many neurologists, nurses and people with MS who have shared their insights and given of their time to help shed some light on the the challenges and mysteries of multiple sclerosis.

ABOUT THE AUTHOR

Steven Manners is the writer/editor of *MSology* (www.msology.ca), a weekly news service for people affected by MS, and *NeuroSens*, a biweekly news service on neurology and psychiatry. For ten years he served as writer/editor of the largest-circulation magazine in Canada for people with MS. Manners is the author of six books, including *Super Pills*, a cultural history of prescription drugs. He lives in Montreal.

www.ingramcontent.com/pod-product-compliance
Lightning Source LLC
Chambersburg PA
CBHW071536200326
41519CB00021BB/6506